MW01124683

SECRETS TO GUT HEALTH FOR WOMEN

HOW PROPER FOODS, EXERCISE, AND STRESS REDUCTION POSITIVELY IMPACT OUR LIFE AND OUR DIGESTIVE SYSTEM

OLIVIA SIMON

© **Copyright 2022 - All rights reserved.**

The content contained within this book may not be reproduced, duplicated or transmitted without direct written permission from the author or the publisher.

Under no circumstances will any blame or legal responsibility be held against the publisher, or author, for any damages, reparation, or monetary loss due to the information contained within this book, either directly or indirectly.

Legal Notice:

This book is copyright protected. It is only for personal use. You cannot amend, distribute, sell, use, quote or paraphrase any part, or the content within this book, without the consent of the author or publisher.

Disclaimer Notice:

Please note the information contained within this document is for educational and entertainment purposes only. All effort has been executed to present accurate, up to date, reliable, complete information. No warranties of any kind are declared or implied. Readers acknowledge that the author is not engaged in the rendering of legal, financial, medical or professional advice. The content within this book has been derived from various sources. Please consult a licensed professional before attempting any techniques outlined in this book.

By reading this document, the reader agrees that under no circumstances is the author responsible for any losses, direct or indirect, that are incurred as a result of the use of the information contained within this document, including, but not limited to, errors, omissions, or inaccuracies.

CONTENTS

No disease that can be treated by diet should be treated by any other means.

— MAIMONIDES

INTRODUCTION

You probably have heard that the road to a healthier you go through a healthier gut. But how do you apply this in real life? Chances are that you know a few diets and supplements that work well for the gut, but are they safe for you? How would you rate your gut health on a scale of 0-10—good, bad, or awful?

Before you answer how you would rate your gut health, let me state some facts about gut health:

- Around 70 million people in the United States are affected by gut health issues.
- About 72% of women experience gut health issues (Laurence, 2017).
- Gut health does not only stay within the abdomen, but is related to many other health

issues including stress, mental health issues, and ADHD.

- Gut health issues can bother anyone at any age, but those nearing their midlife are more likely to have such problems.

I needed to share these facts because many people will deny their gastrointestinal issues until it is too late, and they develop more severe health issues. However, the good news is that most gut offenders are controllable simply by choosing the healthier option while eliminating the bad.

Your gut health doesn't only affect your physical health. It affects your mental and emotional health, making your social life suffer. It's hard to go out with friends when you are feeling sick or worried about how the food you might eat will make you feel.

I understand the struggle you are going through, as I have had gastrointestinal issues throughout my life. It wasn't until I started to make essential changes to my life that I learned everything I needed about my gut health. Throughout this book, you will learn everything about your gut's health and its connection to your brain and other areas of your health. If you are experiencing gut health issues, it's essential to try to make the right changes, but do you know what these changes are? By the end of this book, you will learn all the secrets to regaining your gut health.

1

THE GUT ARCHITECTURE AND FUNCTION

Your gut health is essential to your overall well-being, and in recent years, the importance of your gut has started to fall into the spotlight of professions. Gut health and gut problems are rising, but do you know what your gut is? Some people might think that it is just slang for your stomach or other parts of your digestive system, but simply put, your gut is a collection of organs that constitute about 80% of the immune system and overall health. To improve and maintain your gut health, you must first understand it. In this chapter, we will look at all the aspects of your gut to better understand its structure and the signs that your gut health might be on the decline.

THE HUMAN DIGESTIVE SYSTEM

The common belief that your gut is just your stomach comes from the fact that the stomach is one part of it. Your gut encompasses your entire digestive system. As you know, the digestive system is essential to our lives because it allows us to consume food, absorb nutrients, and remove waste. The digestive system comprises numerous organs, including the GI (gastrointestinal) tract, liver, gallbladder, and pancreas. The GI tract contains "the mouth, esophagus, stomach, small intestine, large intestine, and anus" (Cleveland Clinic, 2021). All these organs are classified as hollow because they allow food to travel from your mouth to your anus.

Unlike plants, which use photosynthesis, or the process of turning sunlight into energy, humans require food as the digestive tract breaks down food, absorbs nutrients from the food, and turns this into energy. When the body absorbs all the nutrients it can from food, the digestive system transports the solid waste for removal, allowing it to repeat the process and energize the body.

The gut makes up nearly 80% of the immune system, essential for absorbing nutrients from the liquids and foods we consume. We do not absorb nutrients externally in large enough doses to sustain us; thus, the digestive tract allows the body to get the nutrients and energy it needs to maintain our health, growth, and cell repair. Nutrients the digestive tract needs to absorb include fats, carbohydrates, proteins, minerals, and vitamins. Water is also essential for the digestive tract and overall health.

The Gut Anatomy

There are many moving parts to the digestive system, all essential to processing nutrients and waste removal. Although we understand that we eat, digest food, and then expel waste, there is a lot more that goes on in our gut, and understanding the different organs and their purpose can help you to pinpoint which areas of your gut are on the decline. All these different organs need to be healthy for your gut and overall health to be good. Here are essential organs that make up our gut anatomy and their purpose.

The Esophagus

The esophagus is the fibromuscular tube that allows food to travel from the mouth and pharynx to the stomach. This tube is approximately 25 centimeters in length. The three muscular layers of the esophagus contract rhythmically to allow food to travel. The hardening of these muscular layers can impact someone's ability to swallow. Another essential part of the esophagus is the upper and lower esophageal sphincter, which prevents gastric reflux and air from entering the esophagus. As its name suggests, the upper esophageal sphincter is at the top of the esophagus and prevents air from entering. The lower esophageal sphincter is at the bottom and prevents your stomach contents from splashing into your esophagus.

The Stomach

After the food has traveled through the esophagus, it enters the stomach. The stomach is known as an intraperitoneal digestive organ that is located in the epigastric and umbilical regions. However, the exact anatomy of a person's stomach can differ in terms of shape, size, and position. There are four different areas of the stomach, including:

1. **Cardia:** at the T11 level and surrounds the superior opening of the stomach
2. **Fundus:** the upper portion of the stomach that is filled with gasses
3. **Body:** the central and largest part of the stomach
4. **Pylorus:** the area where the stomach connects to the duodenum

The stomach also has two sphincters known as the inferior esophageal and pyloric sphincters. The inferior esophageal sphincter allows food to pass from the esophagus into the stomach. The pyloric sphincter separates the pylorus and the duodenum and controls the release of gastric acid and food, also known as chyme, from the stomach. This sphincter constricts itself to stop the release of stomach contents into the duodenum. Gastric pressure builds until, eventually, it pushes through the resistance of the pyloric sphincter.

The Small Intestine

After food leaves the stomach, it enters the small intestine, which consists of the duodenum, jejunum, and ileum. The small intestine is 6.5 meters in length and is essential for the digestion of food and the absorption of nutrients. The duodenum is connected to the pylorus of the stomach and extends to the duodenojejunal junction. There are four parts to the duodenum:

1. **Superior:** called the cap and connected to the liver.
2. **Descending:** contains the major duodenal papilla, an opening for pancreatic secretions and bile.
3. **Inferior:** crosses over the aorta, and inferior vena cava.
4. **Ascending:** connects to the jejunum at the duodenojejunal flexure.

The jejunum and ileum are in the lowest parts of the small intestine and, unlike the duodenum, are connected to one's posterior abdominal wall. There is no distinct point where the jejunum starts and the ileum ends, but their structure differs. As food moves through the small intestine, it continues to be digested, and nutrients are extracted and absorbed.

The Cecum

The cecum is a part of the large intestine and connects the ileum and colon. The cecum is a reservoir for chyme which is released by the ileum. The ileocecal valve connects the ileum and cecum. The ileocecal valve prevents reflux from the large bowel. The cecum used to have a larger purpose in our digestion as it was essential for cellulose digestion, but this is no longer the case for humans now.

The Appendix

The appendix is connected to the end of the large intestine and cecum. The appendix can cause many health issues, including appendicitis, but research has not been able to find any vital functions of this organ. The organ also contains a lot of lymphoid tissue. The position of the appendix's free end can differ in people, including:

- **Pre-ileal:** positioned at one or two o'clock and is anterior to the terminal ileum.
- **Post-ileal:** positioned at one or two o'clock and posterior to the terminal ileum.
- **Sub-ileal:** positioned at three o'clock and parallel with terminal ileum.
- **Pelvic:** positioned at five o'clock and descends over pelvic brim.
- **Subcecal:** positioned at six o'clock and below the cecum.
- **Paracecal:** positioned at 10 o'clock and aligns with the cecum's lateral border.
- **Retrocecal:** positioned at 11 o'clock and is behind the cecum. This is the most common position for the free end of one's appendix.

The Colon

The colon is another organ encompassed in the large intestine and connects the cecum and anal canal. By the time food reaches the colon, it has been digested, and while in the colon, water and electrolytes are absorbed, and the digested food is formed into feces. All necessary nutrients, vitamins, and minerals have been absorbed. The colon forms an arch encircling the small intestine. The colon is 150 centimeters long and can be broken up into four sections:

- **Ascending colon:** the very beginning of the colon and forms the right colic flexure when it makes a 90-degree turn at the right lobe of the river
- **Transverse colon:** goes from the right colic flexure and extends to the spleen. At the spleen, it also creates a 90-degree turn downward, forming the left colic flexure
- **Descending colon:** moves toward the pelvis and turns into the sigmoid colon when it turns medially
- **Sigmoid colon:** makes up about 40 centimeters in length and is in the lower left part of your abdomen

The colon also contains paracolic gutters which are two spaces that lie between the posterolateral abdominal wall and ascending and descending colon. These structures release infected and inflamed material from abdominal organs to collect in areas where it won't disrupt digestion.

The Rectum

The rectum is the lowest part of the lower intestine and stores fecal matter temporarily until it is time for the body to expel them. The rectum connects the sigmoid colon and anal canal. The rectum has two major flexures: the sacral and anorectal flexure. The sacral flexure follows the sacrum and coccyx curve, and the anorectal flexure varies on the tone of your puborectalis muscle. The anorectal flexure plays a big part in fecal continence.

The Anal Canal

The final part of the digestive system and GI tract is the anal canal, which is essential to releasing fecal matter and maintaining fecal continence. As with other parts of the GI tract, there are sphincters within the anal canal that cause it to collapse, except when a person is defecating. The anal canal has both internal and external sphincters. The inner anal sphincter is a thickening of involuntary muscle in the bowel wall and surrounds approximately two-thirds of the anal canal. The external anal sphincter is a voluntary muscle that overlaps slightly with the inner anal sphincter, taking up the lower two-thirds of the anal canal.

EFFECTS OF AGING ON THE GUT

As we age, our bodies go through numerous changes; depending on our lifestyles, the changes and effects of aging can worsen. However, it's important to remember that even if you are the healthiest person you know, you can still see the effects of aging on your gut.

The digestive system is vital and serves to reserve the energy and nutrients we need. This ability to reserve allows the GI system to be shielded from the effects of aging. This means that while other parts of your health and body might see the effects of aging, it can take a while for your gut to start seeing them. However, this doesn't mean you won't see these effects. It is estimated that someone who is gut healthy is likely not to see any effects of aging on their gut before the age of 65 (Mayfair Diagnostics, 2019).

The effects of aging on your gut will likely not affect the entire digestive system or GI tract. Rather, certain parts will be affected. Common changes someone might experience to their gut from aging include:

- **Mouth:** This includes difficulty chewing and swallowing, from decreased bite force to less saliva.
- **Esophagus:** The upper esophageal sphincter tension decreases, and strength reduces in esophageal contractions.
- **Stomach:** There can be an increased risk of ulcers from elasticity changes in the stomach lining. This loss of elasticity makes the stomach more susceptible to damage.
- **Small intestine:** One might see an increased risk of intolerances to food, such as lactose,

when lactase levels decrease. Increased growth of harmful bacteria can reduce the absorption of nutrients, including iron, calcium, and vitamin B.

- **Large intestine:** Movements of contents can start to slow.
- **Rectum:** Decreased contractions cause the rectum to fill too much, leading to constipation.

Acid reflux and constipation are some of the most common first signs that you are experiencing age-related changes to your gut. As we age, we can become more susceptible to these changes, which lead to health issues. However, making the right changes to your diet and lifestyle will help to reduce this risk. Throughout this book, you will learn how to maintain your gut health.

ROLE OF YOUR GUT

The first 1000 days of someone's life are pivotal to our gut health and overall well-being. Healthy development of the gut has been linked to overall health. The gut is home to 100 trillion microorganisms known as microbiota, which aid in food digestion, nutrient and vitamin absorption, and waste removal. Microbiota and gut health also influence the development of our immune systems. People with poor gut health are more likely to have decreased immune functions, as the gut is an essential part of the immune system.

You might know that the brain communicates with the entire body, but there is a vital connection between the gut and the brain. The gut and brain communicate with one another to tell us when we are full or tell the brain that there is something wrong. This triggers the immune system to act.

As we grow, the digestive system and GI tract undergo substantial structural changes in our early lives. There are trillions of microbiota in our guts, but the right composition of these microbiotas must also be to ensure our gut health is good. Imbalances in gut bacteria can lead to poor gut health throughout one's life and poor overall health. Numerous factors can influence this, including the use of antibiotics, the mother's diet during pregnancy, gestational age, mode of delivery, and nutrition.

SIGNS YOUR GUT IS FACING SOME TURBULENCE

Our guts are incredibly complex, and there are numerous reasons someone might have issues with their gut. You might expect that the symptoms of declining gut health would all involve your gut or digestive tract, but this would be false. Declining gut health can cause mental, physical, and emotional symptoms, which you might at first consider to be related to your gut health. Here are some of the signs that your gut health might be on the decline:

- **Upset stomach:** This is a prominent symptom as your stomach is an essential organ in the gut and is where digestion begins. Upset stomachs can be caused for numerous reasons, whether you ate something bad or might be experiencing intolerance to certain foods. Common symptoms include gas, discomfort, bloating, diarrhea, heartburn, constipation, and nausea.
- **Fatigue and tiredness:** Gut microbiota imbalances can cause issues converting food into energy and absorbing nutrients, leading to chronic fatigue.
- **Trouble sleeping:** Insomnia or other sleep disorders can be caused by poor gut health. Poor gut health symptoms such as heartburn and upset stomachs can make it harder to fall asleep and stay asleep. Sleep is essential for maintaining gut health as it can help to regulate

gut microbiota, and poor gut health can disrupt sleep.

- **Intolerance of some foods:** Microbiota imbalances or poor overall gut bacteria cause food intolerances. Intolerances make it harder to digest food and can result in nausea, diarrhea, abdominal pain, gas, and bloating.
- **Extreme food cravings, especially for sugar:** Increased sugar levels are linked to increased inflammation in the body and bad gut bacteria. The high levels of harmful gut bacteria lead to increased cravings, especially for sugary foods.
- **Skin irritations:** Although not all skin irritations are caused by your diet and gut health, eczema, acne, and psoriasis have been shown to be impacted by gut health.
- **Frequent headaches and migraines:** The brain and gut communicate, and poor gut health can cause issues such as migraines and headaches. Nausea and vomiting during migraines, especially, are signs that your gut health is declining. Studies have shown that people who frequently experience headaches and migraines are more prone to gut health issues (Frederick Health, 2021).
- **Autoimmune problems:** Our guts are tightly linked to our immune system, and poor gut

health can cause an increased amount of inflammation. Chronic inflammation triggers the immune system when it's not needed and can lead to autoimmune disorders or when the body attacks its own healthy cells. Common autoimmune problems caused by poor gut health include rheumatoid arthritis, thyroid issues, type 1 diabetes, and multiple sclerosis.

- **Frequent mood changes:** The communication between the gut and the brain and the connection between mental, physical, and emotional health has our emotional and mental health impacted by one's gut health. Inflammation, especially to the nervous system, has been shown to increase one's risk of anxiety and depression. More on how your gut health affects your mind and body will be talked about in the next chapter.

Our gut and its health are complicated, but it is essential to our overall health. It encompasses multiple organs that can be impacted by other health issues. There are trillions of microorganisms in our gut that aid in the digestion, absorption, and removal of waste. Our gut is essential to giving us energy and getting us through the day. Our overall health and immune system rely on our gut, as 80% of the immune system comprises multiple organs in the GI tract. Our gut can be affected by age, but the lifestyle you live now can help to reduce these changes. Throughout this book, we will discuss how your gut affects numerous areas of your life and how you can ensure your gut remains healthy. In the next chapter, we will focus on the impact the gut can have on one's mind and body.

2

HOW YOUR GUT AFFECTS YOUR MIND AND BODY

Although the primary purpose of our gut is to digest food, convert food into energy, absorb nutrients, and remove fecal matter, this is not the only process in which the gut takes part. The gut influences many different processes and areas of the body. Throughout this book, we will focus on numerous ways our gut affects our mind and body, including the gut-body connection, the gut-brain connection, how your gut influences hormones, heart health, and inflammation, and COVID-19 and gut health.

THE GUT-BODY CONNECTION

There is a saying that you are what you eat, and this is very accurate. Your diet is essential to your health, both overall and at a molecular level. As we discussed in the last chapter, developing your gut in your early years is critical for your overall health. However, you can have healthy gut development in your early years, but a poor diet throughout your life can cause many issues with your immune system and inflammation. The link between your gut, diet, immune system, and overall health comes from the gut-body connection.

How the Gut Affects Your Immune System

We touched briefly in the last chapter about how your gut can impact your immune system, as it makes up about 80% of it. Remember that your gut deals with all processes involving food consumption, digestion, mineral and vitamin absorption, and waste removal. When one of these functions is impacted in some way, it can also affect your immune system. This is because our immune system and gut have a symbiotic relationship. The types of food that we eat feed the bacteria in our gut, which helps strengthen or weaken the immune system. However, not all the foods we eat have the same effect on our gut bacteria. Some food will help to fuel the beneficial microbiota, while others will fuel the harmful bacteria. Depending on which types of food you are eating regularly, it can cause an imbalance in the gut microbiota and issues with our immune systems. It's important to remember that within our bodies, our cells and the bacteria inside of us live in close proximity and have developed a symbiotic relationship.

The gut is where the microbiota and the immune system meet and interact. Let's use the example of having an ulcer in your stomach. Your gut and the bacteria inside of it will communicate with your immune system to say that there is a problem that activates the immune system. It's essential to note that the immune system is in charge of keeping the entire body and is influenced by our physical, mental, and emotional health. Let's review the basic functions of our immune system to get an idea of just how important it is and how the gut and its microbiota can influence it.

How Gut Microbiota Affects the Immune System

As we know, trillions of bacteria live in the gut, but when we think of bacteria, we often don't think it would be good for our health. However, studies have revealed that certain bacteria in the gut serve as microbial mediators that help regulate the immune system (Pesheva, 2021). It was only in the last couple of decades that the connection between gut microbiota and the immune system was discovered. The concept of holobiont, or the ecosystem, comprises the human body and the species that live in and around the human body was created to look at how gut microbiota and the cells within the immune system interact and influence one another. The immune system's complexity and gut microbiota formed as human cells and microbiota coevolved together to create a symbiotic relationship within the body. As early as birth, bacteria and our immune system start interacting with one another, as the birth canal has bacteria that help the immune system recognize harmful or healthy bacteria.

As our immune system encounters more bacteria and learns, it strengthens and forms diverse microbiomes within the body. Gut microbiomes also start to form and are essential for immune system strength. The gut microbiome is crucial for developing T-cells, a type of NK cell tasked with distinguishing our cells from foreign bodies. Gut microbiotas are gatekeepers and trainers for these cells. Not all pathogens get recognized; T-cells are essential when this happens because they mediate and destroy infected cells.

Gut health and healthy microbiota signal the body to develop these T-cells, which help boost immune responses. The immune system, in response, populates the gut with healthy microbiota, which maintains the gut and overall health. When gut health is on the decline, immune cells and proteins which live or are produced in the gut are not being produced as much, and the balance of healthy and unhealthy microbiota is thrown off. A lack of immune cells and proteins being produced thus doesn't allow for the gut to signal to the immune system to create as many healthy microbiotas, causing both to decline.

THE GUT-BRAIN CONNECTION

We talked very briefly in the last chapter about the connection between the gut and the brain. One of the most known ways that the brain and gut communicate is by telling us when we are full, but this is one of the many ways that the gut and brain communicate with one another. Think of a time when you were feeling nervous. Did you experience some form of stomach discomfort or nausea? This is because our brain, gut, and mood are extremely connected. Our GI tracts and digestive systems are sensitive to strong emotions such as anxiety, anger, elation, and sadness. Feeling these emotions, especially for an extended period of time, can cause symptoms in our guts. The connection isn't only one way, either. A decline in cognitive abilities or a troubled brain can send signals to our GI tract, especially the stomach and intestines, while a distressed stomach or intestine will also send signals to the brain. The gut-brain connection makes it so that our mood can affect our gut health and vice versa.

Mood and Gut Health

Our nervous system is our body's command center, which allows the brain to send signals throughout the body and controls digestion, movement, thoughts, and breathing, amongst other processes. However, did you know that the gut has a nervous system of its own? This nervous system isn't like our central one as it doesn't think, but it controls digestion, mineral and nutrient absorption, and waste removal. This nervous system is known as the enteric nervous system. The enteric nervous system communicates directly with the brain and can send signals that affect mood. The communication between the gut and the brain is two-way and is both anatomical and physiological. The vagus nerve is essential as it enables the communication between the brain and the gut.

The Gut, Anxiety, and Digestive Problems

Because of the connection our gut and brain have, mental health issues can be the effect of gut health issues or cause them. The gut-brain connection makes it more likely that people who suffer from chronic gut problems such as ulcerative colitis, IBS (irritable bowel syndrome), and Crohn's disease are more likely to experience symptoms of anxiety, depression, or other mental health issues. Our immune system plays a large part in our moods. Think about a time when you were ill. You were likely not in the best of moods, and this is because of the connection our gut and the immune system have to our moods.

Approximately 90% of the body's serotonin produced occurs in the gut. Serotonin is a neurotransmitter that is known as the happy chemical. A healthy gut micro-biome will allow for the proper production of sero-tonin and other neurotransmitters, including dopamine, gamma-aminobutyric acid, and norepinephrine. All of these neurotransmitters are responsible for regulating emotions and triggering feel-ings of anxiety, happiness, and rewards. The produc-tion of serotonin and other neurotransmitters relies on a healthy gut; thus, those that are experiencing some form of gut distress or illness are much more likely to experience anxiety and depression.

Anxiety and depression have also been linked to diges-tive problems. Stomach and intestinal problems such as bloating, heartburn, loose stools, and abdominal cramps are very common physical symptoms of stress which, when experienced chronically, can cause an increased risk of inflammation, anxiety, and depression. The next time you are experiencing stomach or intestinal distress, reflect on what is happening in your life and see what kinds of emotions you are feeling. Are you stressed, anxious, or depressed? This might be a sign that your mental and gut health is on the decline.

Whether your gut health is the cause of declining mental or emotional health, or these negative emotions are the cause of poor gut health, improving your mood can help substantially with your gut health. Here are three ways that you can improve your gut health and boost your mood:

- **Eat fermented foods such as yogurt, miso, kimchi, kombucha, sauerkraut, and kefir.** Fermented foods are full of yeast and bacteria, which act as natural probiotics and aid in improving gut health. They also increase the diversity of gut microbiota.
- **Consume a rainbow of vegetables.** Plants, especially vegetables, are full of dietary fiber that helps break down and digest food. They also produce metabolites such as short-term fatty acids, which help to boost gut health. However, just eating one or two vegetables isn't enough. Different vegetables will produce different metabolites, which will have their

own benefits, which is why eating a variety of vegetables is essential. However, if you have preexisting digestive problems such as IBS, it is crucial to understand which foods, including vegetables, can exacerbate your symptoms.

- **Prioritize sleep and exercise.** Your diet isn't the only factor when it comes to gut health. Your lifestyle also plays a large part in your gut health. Getting enough sleep and exercise is vital for overall well-being. As we sleep, the body can go through automatic processes that enable the immune system to repair and promote diversity within your gut microbiome. Exercise helps to increase endorphins and oxygen flow and triggers the production of short-chain fatty acids that help to boost gut health. It is recommended that adults get seven to nine hours of sleep and 150 minutes of exercise per week

GI SYSTEM AND TOXIN REMOVAL

The body must digest what it consumes to extract nutrients, vitamins, and minerals, but after the body has gotten what it needs, it needs to remove the toxins and waste products left behind. Numerous organs in the GI tract are responsible for toxin removal or detoxing the body, including:

- **Liver:** multiple phases are performed by the liver help to remove toxins, but they depend on the body getting enough nutrients to be completed
- **Kidneys:** the filters of the body that remove toxins from the blood and excrete them through urination
- **Colon:** after the livers and kidneys perform the body's primary detox, the colon physically removes toxins and waste through pooping

Other organs, such as the lungs and skin, also partake in toxin removal but are not part of the GI tract. Lungs remove toxins that are breathed in, while the skin will excrete toxins that cannot go through the colon or bladder, often seen as rashes. When toxins from food and waste products are left in the body, it can lead to deadly consequences.

DIFFERENCES IN WOMEN TOWARD RESPONSE TO NERVE SIGNALS

How the immune system of men and women react to different pathogens, both foreign and self, is inherently different in the innate and adaptive immune systems. Some differences between how women and men respond to different nerve signals are seen as early as birth, but others do not appear until after puberty. Environmental exposures also influence our micro-biomes and how we react to different nerve signals.

Sex-based immunological differences are based on sex and gender, which, although often used interchange-ably in today's age, are very distinct from one another. Sex pertains to someone's chromosomes, sex steroid levels, and reproductive organs. Gender refers to activi-ties and behaviors that are determined by culture and society. Both sex and gender can cause sex-based immunological differences. Genes in the X chromo-some regulate immune function and modulate the sex differences experienced in immune-related diseases.

The differences that sex causes between responses to nerve signals can cause increased frequency, with approximately 80% of people with autoimmune diseases in America being women (Klein & Flanagan, 2016). The treatment of diseases such as cancer are also sex-based, with some treatments being more effective for females versus males. The severity and prevalence of infectious diseases also differ based on sex. Newborn males are more vulnerable to infections and death than newborn females (Klein & Flanagan, 2016). Although there are no definite reasons as to by there are sex differences in how our immune systems work and how we react to different nerve signals, it is theorized that as humans evolved, fundamental mechanisms that increase our ability to reproduce and survive to affect immune responses.

INFLUENCE ON HORMONES

The gut influences our mood and immune system, so it shouldn't be surprising that it can also influence our hormones. The microbiome in our gut influences many aspects of our lives, including the production of many chemicals, bacteria, and cells, within the body. Our metabolism and physiology are tightly linked to our gut, and hormonal balance is a big part of metabolism. Our hormones are vital to our health, with many issues arising from hormonal imbalances, including declining gut health.

Gut-Hormone Connection

The gut-hormone connection is essential because our gut health affects the production and release of hormones. Within our guts is the estrobolome, which is a collection of microbiotas that helps with the metabolizing and release of estrogen. Poor gut health can result in too little or too much estrogen being released, which impacts one's mood, libido, and weight. The microbiome and the gut affect the production of hormones in multiple ways:

- aids in the creation and release of hormones and neurotransmitters such as serotonin, as we talked about in the last section
- promotes the absorption of nutrients, which allows for proper hormone creation
- helps regulate estrogen levels
- boosts the immune system, which further promotes proper hormone levels

Hormones are influenced by several different health factors, including weight, chronic diseases, autoimmune diseases, poor mental health, and poor gut health. Although the creation of estrogen is primarily in the adrenal glands and ovaries, the estrobolome is essential for producing beta-glucuronidase, an enzyme essential for regulating estrogen. This enzyme is also critical for breaking down complex carbohydrates and absorption of flavonoids and bilirubin. The body also metabolizes estrogen, and the waste product afterward has to be dealt with. This occurs in the gut as the liver metabolizes estrogen and delivers it to the gut's bile for excretion. We don't want to reabsorb this estrogen, so a healthy gut and estrobolome help to minimize how much-conjugated estrogen is reabsorbed. A healthy gut will promote the removal of estrogen through urine and stool.

However, poor gut health or gut dysbiosis can result in an imbalance of beta-glucuronidase, which can be created from excess bacteria. This can cause reabsorption of conjugated estrogen resulting in too high estrogen levels. Effects of estrogen dominance include obesity, metabolic syndrome, premenstrual syndrome, infertility, mood disturbance, estrogen-related cancers such as breast and prostate cancer, and heart disease.

Improving your gut health can be a great way to help improve your hormone balance and fortify your gut health for years to come. Improving both can also help to alleviate symptoms of various health issues. Here are some tips to consider for improving your gut health and balancing your hormones:

- **Look at your diet.** As we know, the food we eat plays a large part in bacteria that will be the most active in your diet. Prebiotics and probiotics are great foods to introduce into your diet regularly, and cutting out white carbs such as rice, potatoes, and pasta as much as possible will help to decrease blood sugar levels.

- **Look at your medications.** Regular use of antibiotics disrupts the natural growth of your microbiome, resulting in dysbiosis or the overgrowth of bacteria. However, this change in growth to our microbiota is not permanent, and people usually have natural microbiota growth within six months.
- **Consider your environment.** Estrogen is not only present in our bodies but can also be present in the environment. Phytoestrogens are present in plants, including tofu, soya, and tempeh, which, when consumed, can help to increase estrogen when it is low.
- **Increase your physical exercise.** Detoxification is vital for hormonal balance, and exercising is an excellent way to boost detoxification. Exercising helps to reduce a stress hormone known as cortisol which can adversely impact your hormones.
- **Reduce alcohol consumption.** Everyone has the right to drink alcohol; however, you should understand that it negatively impacts your gut microbiome and the liver. As we know, the liver is responsible for detoxifying estrogen, and the blood and alcohol can cause liver dysfunction leading to more circulating estrogen and estrogen dominance.

GUT HEALTH AND OTHER AREAS OF HEALTH

As we can see, gut health plays a large part in our health, especially with its connection to our immune system and how we absorb nutrients. As we know, there is a saying that we are what we eat, and this is vital as what we put into our guts can have significant consequences on our health, especially long-term. Our gut health can significantly influence our heart health and inflammation, as we have touched on a little bit so far. Gut health is as prominent as ever as inflammation and heart disease are on the rise. But there is also a connection between gut health and COVID-19.

Gut Health and Inflammation

Inflammation is the body's state when the immune system is triggered to respond to a wound, virus, pathogen, or any foreign body. Signs of inflammation will differ depending on what the body is fighting and the health of your immune system. When you fight off a virus or illness, you will likely feel fatigued and want to sleep more. You might also experience body aches and pains. Fever is also very common when someone is fighting off a cold or flu. When you have a wound, the area will be swollen, red, and hot to the touch. The wound that the body is experiencing is not always seen. Inflammation is beneficial for the body when it occurs when needed and not after. Chronic inflammation is when inflammation occurs long after the thing that triggered your immune system is gone. Chronic inflammation can also lead to the development of autoimmune diseases, which have the body attacking its health cells because it perceives them as foreign bodies needing elimination.

The gut's deep connection to the immune system is heavily influenced by the gut microbiome. Imbalances in our gut microbiome make us more susceptible to inflammation and inflammatory disease, including inflammatory bowel disease, heart disease, rheumatoid arthritis, and systemic lupus erythematosus. The foods we eat are highly connected to the amount of inflammation one might experience. Many of the foods people eat in the SAD, such as processed foods and those derived from animals, are connected with higher levels of inflammation. This is because these foods feed opportunistic bacteria within the gut, which then trigger inflammation. The more you eat these foods, the more often you will experience inflammation. Consumption of coffee and alcohol has also been connected to a higher risk of inflammation and inflammatory diseases as coffee feeds the bacteria *Oscillibacter*, which is known for causing IBS. Consumptions of alcohol and sugary drinks are also known to feed unhealthy gut bacteria. Eating a gut-healthier diet is connected to a reduction of inflammation and risk of inflammatory diseases.

Gut Health and COVID-19

With the emergence of COVID-19, we are still discovering the long-term effects of the virus are still being discovered, but there is one discovery that has been made is the possibility of someone developing Long COVID. Long COVID is when someone is experiencing lingering symptoms of COVID months after their initial recovery. These symptoms can include prolonged loss of taste or smell, fatigue, insomnia, and muscle weakness. Although no direct cause of Long COVID has been found, various factors have increased one's likelihood of developing Long COVID.

One of the biggest impactors of whether someone experiences Long-COVID is gut health. In 2020, it was discovered by the Center for Gut Microbiota Research that there are significant changes to our gut microbiomes after catching COVID. COVID-19 is unlike other pathogens the body has faced, and it contains many opportunistic pathogens that feed unhealthy microbiota and reduce the production of healthy microbiota. The disruption to our normal microbiome then causes us to enter into a state of gut dysbiosis, which can become more and more severe in those that are sick. The gut's tie to the immune system makes it so that disturbances can exacerbate symptoms of COVID-19 and result in lingering symptoms.

Studies of people with Long COVID revealed that their gut microbiomes were less abundant and diverse than those of healthy people (Kingsland, 2022). However, not everyone who caught COVID-19 is at risk of developing Long COVID, as many see their gut microbiome returning to normal after recovery. Although there are no set treatments yet for the treatment of disrupted microbiomes, especially connected to Long COVID, theories include changing your diet, taking probiotic supplements, avoiding antibiotics, and fecal microbiota transplants.

Now you know just how important the gut is to our minds and bodies. We often don't understand the importance of eating when we need to and feeding our microbiota the nutrients it needs. Many of the physical, mental, and emotional issues that someone can have can be rooted in poor gut health, and one might see a decrease in symptoms when they make healthy changes to their lifestyle, including eating better, getting enough sleep, and exercising. We have talked a lot about the microbiota and the microbiome already, but what is it really, and how does it affect our bodies? The next chapter will learn about gut microbiota and microbiomes.

3

THE IMMERSIVE WORLD OF GUT MICROBIOTA

Did you know that your gut is a multiverse of bacteria, viruses, and yeast? We have discussed that the gut holds trillions of microbiota, but not all of these are the same. For a healthy gut, there needs to be diversity in our micro-biota, which doesn't always mean they will be good. There is a constant balance between healthy and unhealthy microbiota, which is essential for our gut and overall health. Its resilience and connection to our immune system make you less likely to experience age-related gut health problems until you are around 65 years old. However, when we don't take care of our gut microbiota and microbiome, it makes us more likely to develop gut health issues. We often don't see gut health issues until it is too late. Let's explore microbiota and the microbiome and how they can affect our body and health to better understand the ecosystem living inside us.

GUT MICROBIOTA—AN OVERVIEW

Gut microbiotas are trillions of microbes or bacteria that live within our gut. Although the word bacteria typically have a negative connotation, not all bacteria are harmful, but many are beneficial and essential for our health. It is crucial to recognize that microbiota and the microbiome are different. Microbiota is a broad term encompassing the multiple different types of bacteria, including fungi, microorganisms, and viruses, which are living in one single environment. For example, throughout this book, we talk about the bacteria in the gut or the digestive tract.

The microbiome refers to the entire body and everything that inhabits it, including microbiota, genomes, and external environmental substances. The easiest way to imagine the microbiome is to imagine that your body is a city, and your microbiotas are the citizens. The human microbiome will often refer to the composition of microbiotas and other factors in the body. It is estimated that there are approximately 1,000 species of microbiota within the human body. The levels of microbiotas will differ between people, and certain species of microbiota can live in various parts of the body and vary in their function and levels. When someone has gut health issues, this is likely to mean that they are experiencing an imbalance in their microbiome. When microbiomes are healthy, both unhealthy and healthy microbiotas can co-exist without issues. It is when our microbiomes are imbalanced that we see gut health issues start to arise.

Role of the Microbiota

All microbiota, especially gut microbiota, are essential for living a healthy life, and depending on the species and the location of the microbiota, they will have different roles. Gut microbiota is necessary for the fermentation of endogenous intestinal mucus and dietary fibers, which support "the growth of specialist microbes that produce short-chain fatty acids (SCFAs) and gasses" (Valdes et al., 2018). SCFAs are essential for gut health, with the three main ones produced being:

1. **Acetate:** This is produced the most, and is critical for the growth of other bacteria, as it serves as a metabolite. It also plays a role in central appetite regulation.
2. **Propionate:** It is created in the liver and communicates with gut fatty acid receptors. In

mice, it controls gut hormones and can reduce food intake and appetite.

3. **Butyrate:** This is known for having beneficial effects on energy homeostasis and glucose, along with controlling gut hormones in mice like propionate. Butyrate is essential for maintaining oxygen levels in the gut as well.

The microbiota in our guts is essential, as "there are roughly 10 times more bacterial cells than human cells in the gastrointestinal system" (MacGill, 2022). The microbiota in the gut is responsible for numerous functions, including absorbing nutrients from food, protecting the body from pathogens, helping to regulate the immune system, and boosting biochemical barriers in the intestines and gut. When there is an imbalance in microbiota, the essential functions can be affected, leading to health issues. As we have discussed, multiple things can impact our microbiome, including what we are exposed to as children, genetics, and lifestyles we are having.

Why the Human Microbiota Is Important

The human microbiota is essential for not only one's physical health but also one's overall well-being. When someone is experiencing gut health issues, they can also experience mental and emotional health issues. The same goes the opposite way; however, your mental, emotional, and unrelated physical health issues can cause gut health issues. Imbalance in the gut microbiota has been connected to several health issues, including asthma, celiac disease, diabetes, malnutrition, obesity, heart disease, cancer, autistic spectrum disorder, eczema, and multiple sclerosis.

Your gut microbiota has numerous benefits throughout the body, including nutrition, immunity, behavior, and disease. The primary purpose of gut microbiota is to help digest and absorb nutrients; they are essential for converting food into energy. Foods such as meat and vegetables are made from complex molecules which cannot be broken down and absorbed without the help of gut bacteria. The body cannot absorb plant cellulose without the help of gut bacteria. Your gut's bacteria influence feelings of being full and craving. This is why someone with gut microbiota imbalances will often have extreme cravings and delayed feelings of being full, leading to obesity.

We are exposed to microbes at birth, and in our earliest years, what we consume and are exposed to helps to shape our immune systems and gut health. Early exposure to microbes helps create the adaptive immune system we need to deal with ever-changing bacteria and viruses. Healthy gut microbiota will allow our immune systems to adapt faster and more effectively to fight disease and illness. Our mood and behaviors are linked to our gut health as our microbiota can communicate with our brains. This can be very helpful in boosting mood.

Maintaining a healthy microbiome can help to ensure your overall health and reduce your risk of other diseases. However, it's essential to understand that your microbiota cannot do all the work, and having a healthy gut microbiota does not mean you are not at risk of developing other health issues. Numerous factors, including genetics and the environment, can play a role in the development of health issues.

HOW DOES THE GUT MICROBIOME AFFECT YOUR BODY?

The gut is centered around the food that we eat, but it doesn't only affect our stomachs. The gut microbiome and microbiota, as you now know, are essential to our overall health, and they can affect our bodies and lives in numerous ways. Depending on the composition of your gut microbiome, numerous changes can occur including the development of food sensitivities and changes in your overall health. The gut microbiome and microbiota within it have evolved alongside humans, and with its evolution came changes to how it can affect our bodies. We are exposed to microbes as soon as we are born, and evolution has allowed our microbiomes to diversify and adapt as it encounters new things. As we age, our microbiomes change as well. Diversity in your gut microbiome is essential for all areas of your life. Here are some of the ways that your gut microbiome affects your body:

- **Digesting breast milk and fiber:** Breast milk is the first thing we consume as babies, and the bacteria *Bifidobacteria* grows in babies' intestines to aid in the digestion of breast milk. This species of bacteria absorb the healthy sugars in breast milk and promote proper growth. Fiber is essential for the body, but only certain bacteria can digest it. When fiber is digested, it produces SCFAs, which boost healthy gut microbiota. Fiber is essential to our health as it can prevent heart disease, weight gain, cancer, and diabetes.
- **Helps control the immune system:** We've already discussed how the gut and immune system are connected, but to recap, the microbiota in the gut communicates with the immune system and can influence how the body reacts to different viruses and pathogens.

- **Helps control your brain health:** The central nervous system is connected to the gut as it can communicate and influence one another. The gut's connection to the brain has so that poor gut health can send signals to the brain, leading to poor brain health. Poor gut health can lead to decreased brain function. Many neurotransmitters are produced in the gut, and poor gut health can result in too little or too much of a neurotransmitter being produced, resulting in decreased brain health.

- **Controls blood sugar and lowers your risk of diabetes:** Maintaining your blood sugar levels helps reduce your risk of type 1 and 2 diabetes. Studies have revealed that diverse microbiomes can decrease one's risk of diabetes (Robertson, 2017). The same study also revealed that people experiencing onset type 1 diabetes increased in unhealthy gut bacteria. The bacteria within our guts can also impact our bodies' responses. Another study revealed that people who ate the same food could have different blood sugar levels after eating them because of how their gut bacteria interact with the food (Robertson, 2017).

- **Affect weight:** A balanced microbiome needs to have both good and bad bacteria within it, but they need to be balanced. When there are too many unhealthy microbiotas within the gut, this can increase one's risk of disease and weight gain. Dysbiosis occurs when there is an imbalance of microbiota, which can result in weight gain. The difference in microbiomes is not genetic, as studies of identical twins, one of which was obese and the other healthy, showed a difference in their gut microbiota (Robertson, 2017).

- **Affects heart health:** The microbiome and heart health are both impacted by the foods we eat, and heart health can be affected by the composition of our gut microbiota. Good cholesterol and triglycerides are influenced by gut microbiota as healthy microbiota promote them and help keep heart health up. However, certain bacteria in your gut can also increase your risk of heart disease as they convert certain nutrients, such as choline and L-carnitine, into TMAO, a chemical known for blocking arteries.
- **Affects gut health:** Your microbiome encompasses not only your gut but your entire body, and dysfunctions or imbalances in other parts of the body can impact your gut health. Gut dysbiosis is one of the most common

causes of health issues such as IBS and inflammatory bowel disease. Bloating, abdominal pain, and cramping are often caused by microbes in the gut producing chemicals and gas which irritate the gut. Some species of healthy gut bacteria can prevent disease-causing bacteria from attaching to the intestinal wall, resulting in leaky gut syndrome or other health issues.

How Microbiota Help the Body

The microbiota is essential not only for your gut but for your overall health. Good and bad microbiota present in the body can coexist because they have symbiotic relationships. When these microbiotas are in a symbiotic relationship, the human body, and the microbiota benefit. However, not all of the relationships between microbiota are symbiotic; some are pathogenic, which helps to promote disease. Although there are pathogenic relationships within the body, they are few compared to those that are symbiotic, and a healthy gut can balance these relationships. Disturbances in the gut microbiome result in pathogenic relationships growing, leading to a decline in health and an increased risk of developing health issues. There are numerous causes of disruptions in the gut microbiome, including infectious illnesses, prolonged use of antibiotics, and certain diets.

Our immune systems are our primary defense against pathogens, viruses, illness, and anything dangerous to the health of our bodies. Although it was once believed that cells and microbiota could not communicate, this was proven false as gut microbiota communicates with immune cells to help trigger immune responses. A healthy microbiome helps to protect the body from pathogens and will help to support a stronger immune system. Within our microbiomes, various bacteria prevent the overgrowth of unhealthy and harmful bacteria. Healthy microbiomes will ensure the creation of these vital bacteria and maintain the immune system's balance. Unhealthy microbiomes trigger the immune system more than needed and can lead to autoimmune disorders.

COMPONENTS OF THE GUT MICROBIOME

When we talk about the gut microbiome and microbiota, we are talking about numerous components that all work together to maintain our gut health and overall wellness. We use the term microbiota to describe these components because of the various types and species of microorganisms that live in our guts. There are three main components of the gut microbiome: bacteria, viruses, and yeast.

Bacteria

Bacteria are the most common microbe to live in the gut and body microbiome, which many people mistake as the only component. They are the most abundant in the gut microbiome. Remember that there are trillions of microbiota within the gut and bacteria are neither animal nor plant, and are categorized as single-cell organisms.

Viruses

Although this might seem counterintuitive to our health, our gut microbiome contains viruses. Unlike bacteria, viruses need a host to thrive and multiply. When they don't have a host, they will die off. Not all viruses affect everyone or everything in the same way. This is why humans can catch certain illnesses, but animals cannot. When we think of viruses, we don't often think they are good or healthy, but this isn't the case. Just as there are both good and bad bacteria, there are good and bad viruses within our gut. The healthy viruses serve as protection against damaging bacteria.

Yeast

When we think about yeast, our minds might automatically go to bread because we know it's made with yeast; you might not know that our microbiomes also contain yeast.

Yeast is considered a fungus, and various types live in and out of the body. Candida is the most common yeast that lives within the body. Although this yeast naturally grows in the body, it's essential to limit its growth as it can lead to yeast infections which can occur in the skin, mouth, feet, and private areas. A weak immune system makes you more susceptible to yeast infections. Although yeast can cause infection, foods rich in yeast also have lots of protein and vitamin B, which are essential for our diets. Yeast plays a vital role as it also helps with the absorption of minerals and vitamins. It can also help to fight diseases.

WHAT WIPES OUT GOOD GUT BACTERIA

Although this might be an obvious point to make, we need good gut bacteria for our gut health, physical health, the strength of our immune systems, mental health, and overall wellness. Although it is essential to our lives, people often don't maintain good gut bacteria. There are numerous reasons why this might be the case, including not realizing how daily habits and lifestyle can affect your gut health and not understanding the importance of gut health and bacteria, to begin with. Well, you now know of its significance, but you might not know how just how many things can cause our good gut bacteria to diminish. Here are some of the most common ways that our good gut bacteria are wiped out.

Poor Diet

One of the biggest causes of poor gut health is a poor diet. Our microbiota feeds directly off the food we eat, and when we don't have a diverse range of food feeding our gut microbiota, they cannot thrive. When your diet is poor, it doesn't allow microbiota to recover from harmful substances it might come into contact with, such as antibiotics and infections. You want to ensure that your diet is rich in various nutrients that promote microbiota growth.

Lack of Prebiotics

Prebiotics is a fiber that remains undigested as it travels through the digestive tract and helps promote growth and activity in healthy gut bacteria. A diet that lacks prebiotics won't stimulate enough activity in microbiota, and there will be an imbalance of good and bad. Several foods have prebiotic fiber in them, making it easy to introduce more into your diet. Some foods that are high in prebiotics include oats, bananas, leeks, nuts, onions, garlic, chickpeas, lentils, beans, and Jerusalem artichokes.

Refined Sugars and Artificial Sweeteners

A diet high in sugar and low in fiber does not create an environment for diverse microbiota. Refined sugars have been connected to higher levels of inflammation and stimulate the growth of harmful yeast. Artificial sweeteners, especially those that are non-caloric, although not sugar, are still problematic to the gut. They affect bacteria responsible for weight loss and metabolism, causing many health issues.

Too Much Alcohol

An alcoholic drink from time to time isn't going to cause too much trouble for your microbiota, but consuming too much alcohol can cause damaging effects. Dysbiosis or imbalance in microbiota is very prevalent in alcoholics, leading to many other health issues. The type of alcohol can also impact just how your microbiota is affected. A study revealed that gin actively caused a decrease in healthy microbiota, while red wine had benefits as it increased healthy microbiota (Coyle, 2017).

Antibiotics

Chronic antibiotic use has been shown to have adverse effects on our gut health, despite being used to treat infections caused by many of the bacteria that already live in our bodies. One of the most common is urinary tract infections. Antibiotics work by preventing bacteria from multiplying or killing them together, but they do not only target the harmful bacteria causing the infection. It targets both good and bad bacteria. Antibiotics can also cause a short-term decline in the production of healthy bacteria, leading to a surge of unhealthy ones as a result, even after infections are treated.

Birth Control Pills

Chronic medication use, despite its positive effects on other areas of your life, can cause gut health issues. Birth control pills are hormone-based, and as we know, our hormones are tightly linked to our gut health. Manipulating your hormones through birth control can result in less diversity in your microbiota and disruptions to the functions of specific microbiota.

Lack of Physical Activity

Regular physical activity has many benefits, including boosting gut health. Physical activity is associated with an increased amount of butyrate, an SCFA essential for gut health.

Cigarette Smoking

Tobacco smoke contains thousands of chemicals, including 70 known to be carcinogenic. Smoking cigarettes has been tied to an increased risk of heart disease, lung cancer, Crohn's disease, and inflammatory bowel disease. Smoking decreases gut microbiota diversity, and studies have shown that microbiota starts to diversify when people stop smoking.

Poor Sleep and Not Getting Enough Sleep

When it comes to sleeping, it's essential to ensure the quality of your sleep is good and that you are also getting enough sleep. Just because you have a great five or six hours of sleep, this doesn't mean the body has had enough time to go through all the necessary processes it needs. Getting enough sleep is essential for your gut and overall health. Although there hasn't been a lot of research on the role sleep deprivation has on gut bacteria, preliminary studies have shown it can cause changes in the composition of your gut microbiota.

Too Much Stress

Stress is the silent killer, and it has been linked to numerous different health concerns, including the increased risk of inflammation, diabetes, heart disease, high blood pressure, and many other health concerns.

When under a lot of stress, especially chronically, it affects our microbiome by increasing bacteria that are potentially dangerous for our health, including Clostridium, and reducing beneficial bacteria, such as Lactobacillus.

Pesticides

Not only are the foods we eat, our habits, and our lifestyles a potential risk for our gut microbiome, but external factors can also affect our gut health. Pesticides are one of these external factors. Animal studies have shown that glyphosate, a common pesticide, can have short and long-term effects on our gut microbiome (Nourished by Nutrition, 2019). This pesticide can increase one's gluten intolerance and even lead to celiac disease. It also affects our ability to create amino acids and can inhibit healthy gut bacteria growth.

As you can see from everything we have learned in this chapter and throughout the book, our gut microbiota and gut microbiome are essential for our overall health. When your gut microbiome is healthy and thriving, it can balance all elements, including healthy and unhealthy. However, when we ingest something that isn't good for our microbiota, or there are other health issues at hand, it can cause disruptions in the production and function of our healthy microbiota. When these imbalances are sustained it can lead to various gut health issues. In the next chapter, we will learn about many diseases due to gut dysfunction.

4

GUT DYSFUNCTION

Gut health is essential for our quality of life, but not everyone is blessed with it. You might have gut problems for multiple reasons, including genetics, habits, diet, and environmental factors. It's important to note that although you might be genetically inclined to some more gut issues, this doesn't necessarily mean you will experience them. And the same can go the opposite way. You can have no genetic inclination towards disease and develop it. Also, remember that not all gastrointestinal diseases are also linked to genetics. In this chapter, we will explore what exactly a gastrointestinal disease is, why women are more prone to gut issues, common GI problems women experience, and the warning signs that your gut might be unhealthy.

WHAT ARE GASTROINTESTINAL DISEASES?

Gastrointestinal diseases are any diseases that affect any part of the GI tract: any disease that inflicts any gastrointestinal organs from the mouth to the anus. Regarding gastrointestinal diseases, there are various reasons why someone might develop these, including being genetically inclined, diet, lifestyle, congenital disabilities, and other reasons. Depending on the type of gastrointestinal disease, there might be physical abnormalities in the GI tract causing symptoms. In contrast, others will show no change to the GI tract, but will still experience symptoms. Most gastrointestinal diseases can be prevented and treated. There are two categories of gastrointestinal diseases: functional and structural.

What Are Functional Gastrointestinal Diseases?

Functional gastrointestinal diseases show no apparent change to the structure of any organs of the GI tract, yet someone is still experiencing some form of gastrointestinal symptoms such as diarrhea, vomiting, and bloating. The majority of these types of gastrointestinal diseases occur in the colon and rectum. Movement in the gastrointestinal tract is typically impaired, despite there being no physical change to the structure of the GI tract. Common functional gastrointestinal diseases include constipation, nausea, food poisoning, bloating, gas, diarrhea, GERD, and IBS.

Functional gastrointestinal diseases are typically characterized by the inability to move correctly, resulting in symptoms. There are numerous reasons why someone can experience functional gastrointestinal diseases, including:

- a diet that is low in fiber
- changes in your regular routine or traveling
- stress
- consuming a lot of dairy products
- resisting going to the bathroom
- not getting enough exercise
- taking antacid medications, especially those containing aluminum or calcium
- taking medications such as antidepressants, strong pain medications, and iron pills
- pregnancy
- overuse of anti-diarrheal medications as they weaken our bowel muscles resulting in less motility

What Are Structural Gastrointestinal Diseases?

Structural gastrointestinal diseases are caused when structural changes to the GI tract are visible when examined, and these changes result in the GI tract not working properly. Depending on the structural abnormality, they can be removed or fixed with surgery. Here are some examples of structural gastrointestinal diseases.

Constipation

Constipation can be both functional and structural, as your diet and structural abnormalities can cause it. Constipation is characterized by the inability to have a bowel movement or infrequent bowel movements. Typically, three or fewer bowel movements a week are considered constipation. Usually, constipation is caused by insufficient fiber in one's diet and results in straining, leading to more health issues. Constipation can be treated by increasing water and fiber intake, going to the bathroom when you feel the urge, and getting regular exercise.

IBS

Irritable bowel syndrome, which is also known as irritable colon, nervous stomach, and spastic colon, is characterized by the muscles of the colon contracting more or less than normal. It is considered to be a structural and functional GI disease. Symptoms of IBS include excess gas, changes in bowel habits, bloating, constipation, diarrhea, abdominal cramps, and pain.

Various factors can trigger IBS, including stress, certain foods, and medications. There are various treatments for IBS, and depending on the severity of your IBS, some treatments will work better than others. Common treatments include medication, minimizing stress and learning coping mechanisms, drinking more water, avoiding too much caffeine, increasing fiber intake, avoiding foods that trigger your IBS, and getting enough sleep.

Internal and External Hemorrhoids

Hemorrhoids are structural diseases characterized by swollen blood vessels in your anal canal. They are typically caused by excessive straining when trying to move your bowels. They can occur internally and externally, and they can cause pain. Internal hemorrhoids are when blood vessels of the anal opening fall into the anus and become irritated. They can become so irritated that they start to bleed. They can also become so bad that they prolapse or stick out of the anus. External hemorrhoids occur in the veins under the skin outside of the anus. With too much straining, they can burst, resulting in blood clots that will need surgery to remove. Other treatments for hemorrhoids include improving your bowel habits, considering surgery, and considering ligating bands.

Anal Fissures

Anal fissures are characterized by cracks or split in the lining of the anal opening. The most common cause is a result of hard or watery stools. These cracks cause the muscle underneath the lining to be exposed, which is extremely painful. Symptoms include burning pain, spasms, and bleeding after bowel movements. Treatments include pain medication, increased dietary fiber intake, and sitz baths. Surgery can also be used to repair the lining if these treatments do not work.

Colon Polyps and Cancer

Approximately 130,000 Americans are diagnosed with colorectal cancer yearly (Cleveland Clinic, 2021a). Although there is no direct cause of colon cancer, there are various risk factors that can make someone more at risk of developing cancer. Symptoms of colon cancer include bowel movement changes, blood in and on a stool, abdominal pain, constant tiredness, narrower than normal stool, and weight loss. Early screening is used to help detect signs of cancer and discover it early on so that treatment will have a greater chance of success.

These are just a few examples of structural gastrointestinal diseases, but many more can affect someone. Be sure to contact your healthcare provider if you think you are developing any signs of gastrointestinal distress.

WOMEN ARE MORE PRONE TO GUT ISSUES THAN MEN

Women are more prone to gut health issues than men, with approximately 72% of women have suffered from occasional gut issues, and 64% of these women are unwilling to talk about their gut issues or seek help because of it (Renew Life Probiotics, 2016). But why is this?

Hormonal imbalances are common in women, especially during puberty, and as we know, there is a connection between gut health and hormones. Poor gut health is tied to hormonal imbalances. When these are not corrected, it can lead to gastrointestinal issues to rise. There are numerous reasons on top of gut health issues that can cause hormonal balances and lead to gastrointestinal diseases. Treatment of hormonal imbalance might be able to stop the regularity of these health concerns, but you will also need to seek treatment for gastrointestinal issues.

Stress is highly linked to gut health, as we know, and is even linked to developing ulcers within the GI tract. Stress impacts our entire body, and chronic stress can be especially hard on the gut. Women typically stay more stressed out than men, leading to more stress-related health issues, including gastrointestinal problems.

Common GI Problems in Women

There are no ties between sex and GI problems, but our diets, stress levels, environment, aging, and lifestyles can all play a large part in developing gastrointestinal diseases. Not seeking help when gastrointestinal problems first arise can also impact the severity of one's disease. However, many people don't get the help they need because they write off what they are experiencing as something else or think that it will pass. It's very important to be aware of the common GI problems that you might face, so here are a few common GI problems women have been prone to:

Functional esophageal disorders

- functional heartburn
- functional dysphagia
- chest pain that is assumed to be originating in the esophagus
- globus

Stomach problems

Women have a slower emptying time than men when it comes to their stomach, which can lead to more bloating and nausea. Inflammation of the stomach is also common amongst women as they tend to take more over-the-counter pain medication such as Tylenol or Advil to cope with menstrual cramps, headaches, and other issues. Over time, these medications can cause inflammation of the stomach.

Functional gastroduodenal disorders

- aerophagia
- chronic idiopathic nausea
- rumination syndrome
- cyclic vomiting syndrome
- functional vomiting
- functional dyspepsia

Functional bowel disorders and colon issues

- IBS and IBD
- constipation
- unspecified functional bowel disorder
- diarrhea
- colon cancer

Functional abdominal pain syndrome (FAP)

Liver and small intestine

Women have two enzymes that help to break down medication. This means that women and men can react to different medications, and when this isn't considered, medication can create problems for treatment and cause further damage.

Gallbladder and sphincter of Oddi disorders

Women empty their gallbladders slower than men, which makes them more likely to develop gallstones.

- gallbladder disorder
- pancreatic sphincter of Oddi disorder
- biliary sphincter of Oddi disorder

Functional anorectal disorders

- fecal incontinence
- defecation disorders such as inadequate defecatory propulsion and dyssynergic defecation
- anorectal pain caused by levator ani syndrome and chronic proctalgia
- unspecified functional anorectal pain
- proctalgia fugax

Common problems during pregnancy

Nausea is very common with pregnancy, but it is not the only gut issue that might arise. As a baby grows and pushes on different organs, stomach emptying can be affected. Constipation also occurs during pregnancy, both caused by the growing size of the baby and the increase of hormones such as progesterone, which promote the child's growth. Heartburn is also very common with pregnancy, and there is the old wives' tale that babies with a lot of hair have mothers experiencing more heartburn.

WARNING SIGNS OF AN UNHEALTHY GUT

Gastrointestinal diseases do not just show up out of the blue one day. Typically, many warning signs will tell you that your gut health is taking a turn for the worse. Paying attention to your gut health and seeing the warning signs can prevent you from developing worse gastrointestinal conditions. Taking note of the warning signs will allow you to take control of your gut health and make the improvements you deserve. Here are some warning signs of an unhealthy gut:

- **Upset stomach:** This includes stomach aches, gas, bloating, constipation, diarrhea, and heartburn.

- **A high-sugar diet:** When our microbiota balance is off, we often crave high-sugar foods. This is because sugary and processed foods reduce good microbiota and grow unhealthy microbiota.

- **Unintentional weight loss or gain:** Any sudden or unintentional weight loss or gain can be a sign that there is some form of impairment in your body's metabolism and absorption of nutrients. Weight loss is often tied to the body not absorbing enough nutrients, while weight gain is tied to the development of insulin resistance.

- **Constant fatigue and sleep disturbances:** Sleep is essential to our overall wellness and gut health. Not getting enough sleep can cause decreased gut health, but it can also be a sign. Trying to fall asleep with gut discomfort is challenging, leading to sleep disturbances and being fatigued.

- **Skin irritation:** The bacteria growing in our gut can often create skin problems as poor bacteria grow. Inflammation can also occur, showing redness of the skin. Psoriasis has been tied to gut health.

- **Auto-immune conditions:** inflammation is widespread when someone is experiencing poor gut health and, when left untreated, can lead to the development of auto-immune disorders.

- **Food intolerances:** When someone has a food intolerance, this is because the body has problems digesting it. Food intolerance is typically caused by poor-quality bacteria in the gut and a lack of diversity. You might have food intolerance signs, including gas, bloating, abdominal pain, nausea, and diarrhea.
- **Migraines:** We already know there is a connection between the gut and the brain. It shouldn't be surprising then that poor gut health can cause migraines.
- **Mood swings:** The brain-gut connection can also cause mood swings. Inflammation of the gut can affect our central nervous system, leading to mood swings and other mental and emotional health problems.

Digestion starts in the mouth with chewing and releasing enzymes that begin to break down food. Next time you sit down for a meal, don't just gulp it down— pay attention to what you are eating and slowly swallow the food. Half-chewed food takes more time to get digested and thus puts more load on your gut. When you mindfully eat your food, you will notice that you become fuller faster, and you might not notice as many gut disturbances after eating. When you eat fast and don't thoroughly chew your food, it makes it much harder for your stomach to signal to your brain fast enough to tell you to stop eating, leading to overeating and strain on the gut. When we overeat, we often have stomach pain, bloating, and cramping. Slowing down to take time to eat might allow you to see improvement in your gut health.

Gut dysfunction is very hard to deal with, and the best way to reduce your risk of developing a gastrointestinal disease is to help maintain your gut microbiota. Some gastrointestinal diseases are not always caused by gut microbiota imbalance but can result from structural issues in the GI tract. In the next chapter, we will explore numerous gut problems more in-depth and talk about getting your gut health issues diagnosed.

5

DIAGNOSING GUT PROBLEMS—A CLOSER LOOK AT THE G.I. PROBLEMS

G ut health issues are irritating, yet they are prevalent, and as we learned in the last chapter, women are more prone to them than men for various reasons. Gut problems are not something to be brushed off to the side, and it's essential to be aware of what you might be experiencing and how to deal with them. If you suspect you are experiencing one of the issues we will discuss or any other gut health issues, contact a health care provider and look towards getting diagnosed. This chapter will outline some of the most common gastrointestinal problems people develop.

IRRITABLE BOWEL SYNDROME

IBS is a common GI problem; however, this doesn't make it any less uncomfortable or severe. This disorder affects the large intestine and is categorized as a functional gastrointestinal disease. As a functional disease, a part of the disorder is miscommunication between the brain and the gut. The prevalence of this connection makes it so that IBS symptoms typically are worsened during times of stress, anxiety, and other negative emotions. Approximately 10-15% of American adults have IBS, but only 5-7% have a proper diagnosis (Cleveland Clinic, 2020). People with IBS develop sensitivity in their digestive tract and will see changes in how their bowel muscles contract. A few other names for IBS include spastic colon, irritable bowel, irritable colon, and nervous stomach. Symptoms of IBS include:

- the appearance of bowel movement changes, such as being harder or looser than normal
- changes in the frequency of bowel movements
- cramping
- abdominal pain
- bloating
- excess gas
- alternating between constipation and diarrhea
- mucus in the stool with a whitish appearance.

Many people will have symptoms of IBS, but they will ignore them, saying they just ate something bad or are having a lousy gut day. But getting a diagnosis of IBS and getting treatment for it can help to improve your quality of life. But people will often ignore the signs until it is too late. Seek professional help immediately if you are experiencing any of the following symptoms: sudden weight loss, iron deficiency anemia, difficulty swallowing, persistent pain even after a bowel movement, rectal bleeding, diarrhea, and unexplained vomiting.

There are three types of IBS that people can experience including:

1. **IBS-C (irritable bowel syndrome with constipation):** stools are lumpy and hard most of the time
2. **IBS-D (irritable bowel syndrome with diarrhea):** stools are watery and loose most of the time
3. **IBS-M (irritable bowel syndrome with mixed bowel habits):** both hard and soft stools in a single day

Causes of IBS

There has been no discovery of a direct cause of IBS; various factors play into the development of IBS. IBS is prevalent in people ranging from teenage to their early 40s. Although there is no direct cause of IBS, women are twice as likely to develop it than men. Here are some of the most common causes of IBS.

Family History

IBS is one of the many gastrointestinal diseases with a genetic link. A family history of IBS, especially a close relative such as a parent or grandparent, can increase your likelihood of developing IBS but does not make it a definite possibility.

Nervous System Abnormalities

The nerves in our nervous system are essential for communicating with the brain, and when there are abnormalities, it can result in perceiving more than normal discomfort as your intestinal muscles stretch and contract. Nerve malfunctioning can also react in the body overreacting to normal changes that occur during digestion leading to GI symptoms such as pain and cramping.

Stronger or Weaker Muscle Contractions than Normal

Muscle contractions allow your intestines to move the food throughout the GI tract. Muscles that are too weak can result in hard stools and constipation. Muscles that are too strong can result in bloating, diarrhea, and gas.

Changes in the Composition of Gut Microbiota

Although there is no research on what microbiota might cause IBS, changes in our gut microbiota can make it easier for people to develop IBS.

Severe Infection

Gastroenteritis or diarrhea resulting from a virus or bacteria has been linked to the possible development of IBS. It is theorized that this is connected to the increased harmful bacteria in the intestines associated with an infection or virus.

Stress (Especially From a Young Age):

As we already know, stress is associated with developing many health issues, including IBS. Exposure to a lot of stress, especially from a young age, causes gut health issues such as IBS.

Triggers of IBS

IBS is a gastrointestinal disease that can be treated but can be triggered even with treatment. Avoiding triggers will make IBS much easier to cope with and decrease the amount of strain on your GI tract. The most common trigger for IBS is food. The food that triggers your IBS will depend on the person and any previous intolerances and allergies. You might not have an intolerance to a type of food, but you might notice that it sometimes upsets your stomach more than other foods. Be mindful of what you are eating and how you feel afterward. This can help you determine which foods make you feel bad, and which don't. Be mindful of drinks as well. Common foods that trigger IBS may include cabbage, beans, dairy, carbonated drinks, and wheat.

The second biggest trigger for IBS is stress, anxiety, and depression. Any form of intense emotion, especially negative ones, can be triggering for your IBS. You might notice your symptoms are worse during periods of stress, anxiety, or depression. Learning to cope with stress healthily and manage depression or anxiety can also help manage your IBS.

LEAKY GUT SYNDROME

When someone says Leaky Gut Syndrome (LGS) to a doctor, they might get mixed reactions. Not all doctors think of LGS as being a diagnosable condition. Until recently, LGS wasn't studied much, but the research being conducted as of late points towards LGS being a diagnosable condition that has ties to numerous other medical conditions. LGS affects the lining of our intestines and results in gaps forming in the intestinal wall. These gaps then allow bacteria and toxins to grow to leak from the intestines and into the bloodstream. The intestinal walls naturally have tight openings to allow nutrients and water to enter the intestines. LGS occurs when these openings widen and allow bacteria and toxins to enter the bloodstream.

The limited amount of research on LGS makes it hard to fully understand the impact that it can have on the body, but it is connected to various other health conditions, including IBS, Celiac Disease, Crohn's, diabetes, chronic liver disease, PCOS (polycystic ovarian syndrome), and food intolerances and allergies. Research hasn't been able to conclude whether it is a cause or a symptom of these other conditions. More research must be conducted to determine if LGS might also be linked to depression and anxiety.

The dispute with LGS being a diagnosable condition might also come from the numerous symptoms it shares with other gut problems and whether it is a disease on its own or just another symptom. It shares many symptoms with other diseases and makes it harder to identify without proper examinations. Symptoms associated with LGS include:

- chronic bloating, diarrhea, or constipation
- fatigue
- headaches
- skin problems, including rashes, eczema, and acne that are not normal for you
- joint pain
- confusion
- nutritional deficiencies
- widespread inflammation

Research hasn't shown a direct cause for LGS, but they have found some risk factors that can increase your likelihood of developing it. These factors are associated with gut inflammation and increased intestinal permeability, which makes it easier for things to enter and leave the intestines. Risk factors related to LGS include chronic alcohol consumption, diabetes, stress, autoimmune disorder, frequent infections, and poor nutrition. Poor nutrition is especially associated with LGS, as our microbiota protect the intestinal walls. When we are not getting the nutrients we need, this increases intestinal permeability.

The lack of research associated with LGS makes it much harder to determine the causes and risk factors associated with LGS, but preliminary studies reveal that your lifestyle might play a big part in the development of LGS. Diet and chronic stress are considered to be the most significant factors.

CROHN'S DISEASE

Crohn's disease is one type of inflammatory bowel disease which causes inflammation of the tissue of the digestive tract. The inflammation caused by Crohn's can occur in numerous areas of the digestive tract, but it most commonly occurs in the small intestines. Unlike other gastrointestinal issues, Crohn's is not curable and will be a lifelong disorder once it develops. The inflammation creates irritation in the bowels leading to various symptoms, including:

- abdominal pain
- chronic diarrhea
- rectal bleeding
- fever
- loss of appetite

- anal fissures
- anal fistulas
- weight loss
- abnormal skin tags
- mouth sores

Although Crohn's is an inflammatory bowel disease, people with Crohn's can also experience symptoms outside of the intestines or where the inflammation is occurring. These symptoms include

- inflammation of eyes, skin, joints, bile ducts, and liver
- kidney stones
- delayed sexual development and growth in children
- anemia

Crohn's can be very dangerous, especially if you leave it untreated and do not seek professional help. Whether you have been diagnosed with Crohn's or you, suspect that you have some form of Crohn's or another gastrointestinal disease, make sure you seek professional help immediately if you are experiencing blood in your stool, severe abdominal pain, unexplained weight loss, nausea, vomiting, and fever.

Just like with IBS, there are different types of Crohn's, and they are defined by which part of the GI tract is affected by the inflammation and irritation. There are five types of Crohn's disease include:

1. **Ileocolitis:** This is the most common form of Crohn's disease and affects the terminal ileum, the end of the small intestine, and the colon. Symptoms of this type of Crohn's disease include cramping, diarrhea, significant and sudden weight loss, and pain in the lower right and middle part of the abdomen.
2. **Ileitis:** This affects the ileum and has similar symptoms to ileocolitis, and in severe cases, people can develop inflammatory abscesses or fistulas in the lower right section of the abdomen.
3. **Jejunoileitis:** This occurs in the jejunum or upper part of the small intestine and typically is shown as patchy spots of inflammation. Symptoms include cramps, abdominal pain after eating, and in severe cases, fistulas.
4. **Gastroduodenal Crohn's disease:** This type affects the stomach and duodenum, or the beginning of the small intestine. Symptoms include loss of appetite, weight loss, nausea, and vomiting.

5. **Granulomatous (Crohn's) Colitis:** This occurs
   in the colon and has symptoms such as rectal
   bleeding, diarrhea, skin lesions and joint pains,
   and ulcers, abscess, and fistulas around the
   anus.

Causes of Crohn's Disease

Crohn's can affect anybody, but it has been shown that
it is extremely prevalent in people aged 15-35. The
exact causes of Crohn's disease are unknown; however,
research has been able to determine two factors that are
linked to Crohn's disease and might be leading causes
of the development of Crohn's disease. The first leading
cause that has been found is one's immune system. Our
immune system, as we know, is triggered to help fight
off bacteria and viruses. It is theorized that Crohn's
might be caused by someone's immune system being
triggered to the GI tract because of bacteria, and atyp-
ical responses or inflammation can result in our
immune system starts to attack our healthy cells, thus
damaging the GI tract and leading to the development
of Crohn's disease.

The second leading cause that scientists have found is
genetics. Studies looking at people with Crohn's disease
revealed that it is much more common among family
members, with approximate 5-20% of people with any

form of irritable bowel disease having a parent, sibling, or child that also has an irritable bowel disease (Crohn's and Colitis Foundation, 2019).

Risks Associated with Crohn's Disease

On top of a family history of Crohn's and your immune system, various risk factors can increase your likelihood of developing Crohn's disease. These risk factors will not be the sole cause of your Crohn's disease, but when paired with the potential causes discussed in the previous section, they will increase your risk of developing Crohn's. Risk factors associated with Crohn's include:

- **Ethnicity**: Crohn's disease can affect anyone of any race or ethnicity, but studies have revealed that Caucasians, mainly from Eastern Europe, are the most at risk of developing Crohn's (Mayo Clinic, 2020). However, Crohn's has increased in various communities, including African Americans and Middle Eastern individuals.
- **Age**: Although Crohn's can occur at any age, those between 15-30 are most at risk of developing the disease.
- **Cigarette smoking**: This is one of the controllable risks associated with Crohn's and

has been connected to a more severe version of the disease.

- **Nonsteroidal anti-inflammatory medication use**: These medications are over-the-counter pain medications, such as Advil and Tylenol, which can cause inflammation in the bowl after prolonged use and increase your risk of Crohn's.

Complications With Crohn's Disease

Crohn's is a lifelong disease, and with that can come many health complications, especially if you are not maintaining your Crohn's well and are actively eating foods that can irritate it, you can develop numerous complications. Complications can also arise even if you take care of yourself, watch what you eat, and seek professional help when you notice changes. Here are some of the most common complications that can arise with Crohn's disease:

- **Malnutrition:** Crohn's disease occurs in the intestines, a primary area for digestion and nutrient absorption. Crohn's, especially severe cases, can make it very hard to eat because of the pain, cramping, discomfort, and diarrhea, and the inflammation of the intestines makes it harder to absorb nutrients, leading to malnutrition.

- **Bowel obstructions:** The thickness of the intestinal walls can be affected, as Crohn's can scar the bowel, causing it to be narrow—which over time can increase the risk of bowel obstructions, as digested food cannot make its way through the intestines.
- **Anal fissures:** These small tears of the tissues around the anus can often occur with Crohn's, especially when someone is straining with hard stools.
- **Fistulas:** Fistulas are abnormal connections between body parts, and Crohn's often occurs between the intestine and abdominal wall. These can lead to abscesses and infections and, when left untreated, can be life-threatening.
- **Ulcers:** These are open sores that can occur anywhere in the digestive tract. The chronic inflammation associated with Crohn's increases the likelihood of ulcers.
- **Colon cancer:** As is the nature of Crohn's, the colon is heavily impacted and can increase one's likelihood of developing colon cancer. Regular colonoscopies can help detect colon cancer earlier and increase treatment success.

- **Skin disorders:** Hidradenitis suppurativa is common amongst people with Crohn's and can create deep nodules, abscesses, or tunnels forming in various parts of the body, including the groin, armpits, genital area, and under the breasts.
- **Blood clots:** Crohn's has been shown to increase the risk of developing blood clots.
- **Medication risks:** Immune-system-blocking medication is often used to treat Crohn's, which comes with various risks, including infection, skin cancers, and lymphoma. Corticosteroids are also linked to numerous health issues, including high blood pressure, bone fractures, cataracts, diabetes, and glaucoma.

ULCERATIVE COLITIS

Ulcerative Colitis is an inflammatory bowel and autoimmune disease that affects the large intestine primarily. This condition, like Crohn's, is a lifelong condition with the immune system attacking the intestine wall and injuring the bowel. Inflammation is prominent in Ulcerative Colitis and typically begins in the rectum and can travel into the colon. Irritation and open sores develop within the large intestine, which causes pain and bleeding to occur.

The severity of someone's Ulcerative Colitis will depend on the area impacted and the treatment that someone is receiving. How much inflammation you have and the severity of it will differ for everyone. You might have severe inflammation, but it's only impacting a small area, or you can have a large area affected by mild inflammation.

Ulcerative Colitis is a lifelong condition; however, there are often periods that someone will go through which they have little to no symptoms. This is called a remission period. There will also be times when someone has a flare-up, or the disease is in an active state. Treatment and therapy for Ulcerative Colitis aim to keep someone in a remission state for as long as possible.

The development of this disease typically occurs between the age of 15-30, just like Crohn's disease. However, after 30, it is possible to develop this disease, with chances decreasing between the ages of 50-70. This disease affects women and men equally. Approximately 50% of the people diagnosed with Ulcerative Colitis have mild symptoms, and there is an increased risk of arthritis, liver disease, osteoporosis, and inflammation in other body parts, especially the eyes (Cleveland Clinic, 2020a).

There are a few symptoms that might give you a hint that your gut health is taking a turn for the worse, and you might be developing Ulcerative Colitis. These early symptoms include diarrhea, fatigue, abdominal cramping, anemia, weight loss, and nausea. If you are experiencing any of these early signs, contact your doctor. If you do not seek treatment or professional help, other symptoms can arise, including:

- blood, pus, and mucous in stool
- fever
- severe cramping
- joint pain
- mouth sores
- loss of nutrients and fluids
- liver disease

Types of Ulcerative Colitis

All types of Ulcerative Colitis involve the rectum and large intestine; however, how much is affected will determine the type of Ulcerative Colitis someone has. The first type that someone can develop is *ulcerative proctitis*, which has inflammation occurring in the rectum and the lower portion of the colon. The second type of Ulcerative Colitis is known as *pancolitis*, which has the entire large intestine affected. *Limited or distal colitis* is the third type of Ulcerative Colitis, with only the left side of the large intestine affected by the disease.

Causes of Ulcerative Colitis

Much like with Crohn's disease, researchers haven't been able to pinpoint the exact cause of ulcerative colitis, but there are various theories. Because Ulcerative Colitis is an autoimmune disease, the immune system is theorized to be the main cause of the development of Ulcerative Colitis. Although it isn't understood why the immune system is triggered to attack cells within the intestines, the immune system attacking itself leads to inflammation and wounds. It is theorized that a combination of genetics and environmental factors increases the likelihood of someone developing Ulcerative Colitis. Like Crohn's, approximately 20% of people diagnosed with Ulcerative Colitis have a family member who also has the disorder (Cleveland Clinic, 2020a).

Anyone can develop Crohn's, but factors that can increase your likelihood of developing the disease include:

- eating high-fat diets
- frequent use of nonsteroidal anti-inflammatory drugs (NSAIDs) being of European or African descent.

Complications Associated With Ulcerative Colitis

People who are receiving treatment for their Ulcerative Colitis and being mindful of their triggers will likely not experience complications because of their disease; however, they are still possible. The less care you put into taking care of yourself will increase your chance of complications. Common complications associated with Ulcerative Colitis include:

- increased risk of bowel cancer
- damage to the bile ducts in the liver, also known as primary sclerosing cholangitis
- poor development and growth in children and young adults

Triggers of Ulcerative Colitis

Ulcerative Colitis comes with active and remission periods that involve someone's disease being triggered, which has someone actively experiencing symptoms or periods of remission where they do not experience any symptoms. The triggers of someone's Ulcerative Colitis will be different for everyone, but here are the most common triggers for flare-ups:

- **Emotional stress:** As we have learned, our health is tightly linked to stress, and your

SECRETS TO GUT HEALTH FOR WOMEN | 103

Ulcerative Colitis can be triggered by any form of stress, especially emotional stress. Learning to cope with your stress healthily and practice healthy habits will help to manage your Ulcerative Colitis.

- **Antibiotics:** Antibiotics do not only target harmful bacteria. They kill or disable positive bacteria's ability to grow and function, leading to the risk of flare-ups.
- **Medication use:** NSAIDs, although helpful for the moment when it comes to relieving yourself of pain, have negative impacts on your intestinal health and cause flare-ups.

Your diet is essential when it comes to dealing with Ulcerative Colitis. Although your diet isn't going to cause the development of this disease like it does others, it can cause flare-ups and also worsen the severity of your symptoms. The foods that trigger your Ulcerative Colitis will be different for everyone, and to find out what yours are, write down what you are eating and then reflect on how it made you feel. Here are some of the most common problem foods:

- foods and drinks high in sugar
- carbonated drinks
- alcohol

- dairy products
- salt
- greasy foods
- high-fiber foods

CONSTIPATION

There is often the common misconception that constipation is when you cannot poop for a long time, but
constipation occurs when you have three or fewer
bowel movements per week. Although how often
someone produces a bowel movement will be different
for everyone, the definition of constipation is three or
fewer bowel movements a week. The longer time
passes between bowel movements, the harder it
becomes to have a bowel movement. Three characteristics of constipation include:

- painful and difficult to pass bowel movements
- feeling like your bowels aren't empty after
  using the bathroom
- dry and hard stools

Constipation is one of the most prevalent gastrointestinal problems that people experience—approximately 2.5 million people a year go to the hospital or
doctor with complaints of constipation (Cleveland

Clinic, 2019). Constipation is so common because how it occurs is not tied to disease but can be linked to various factors. Constipation occurs when the body absorbs too much water from stool which causes it to harden and dry out, making it harder to pass. Water needs to be absorbed from digested food to create a solid stool, but too much water being taken out will lead to constipation.

Constipation can occur as a one-off, where you become constipated, get treated, and never experience it again, or maybe just once or twice more. Or you can develop chronic constipation, which has you experiencing constipation regularly. Whether you experience constipation only a handful of times in your life, or you experience it chronically, the symptoms will be the same:

- You have three or fewer bowel movements per week. However, it's important to remember that your bowel movement habits can differ, and you might usually only go to the bathroom twice a week.
- Stools are challenging to pass and painful.
- Stools are hard and dry.
- You feel nauseous and bloated.
- You're experiencing cramps and stomach aches.
- You feel sluggish.

Fecal impaction is a condition that results from constipation that is not treated, so here are some symptoms to look out for:

- abdominal pain, especially after eating
- headache
- nausea and vomiting
- persistently feeling like you have to use the bathroom but then being unable to
- weight loss and poor appetite
- liquid stool, which is not diarrhea and is caused by stool leaking around the impaction

When not treated, fecal impaction can also lead to rapid pulse, dehydration, fever, agitation, breathing, urinary incontinence, and confusion.

Causes of Constipation

Unlike some of the other gastrointestinal problems we have discussed, doctors know many reasons why someone might be experiencing constipation. There are essentially three categories that the causes of constipation can fall into, and these include habits and lifestyles, medical conditions, and medications.

Causes of constipation that involve our habits and lifestyles include:

- low-fiber diets
- living a sedentary lifestyle or not getting enough exercise
- experiencing chronic stress and burnout
- resisting the urge to go to the bathroom, such as not liking using public bathrooms
- changes to your routine, such as a sudden change in diet, traveling, and not having a constant sleep schedule
- eating a lot of cheese and milk
- not drinking enough water

Everyone will react differently to these possible causes, as some people are more prone to becoming constipated or become constipated easily, or maybe their guts are more resistant to constipation. No matter how resistant you feel you are to constipation, it is best to avoid these habits and lifestyles, which can increase your risk of becoming constipated.

Medical conditions which are linked to constipation include:

- colorectal cancer
- diverticular disease

- irritable bowel syndrome
- pregnancy
- outlet dysfunction constipation, which is a defect in the pelvic floor muscles that affect the coordination of muscles that support the lower abdomen and pelvis, and plays a role in the release of stool
- endocrine problems, including diabetes, hypercalcemia, underactive thyroid gland, and uremia
- lazy bowel syndrome, which has the large intestine weakly contracting and retaining stool
- bowel disease, including lupus, amyloidosis, and scleroderma
- structural defects in the gastrointestinal tract, including the imperforate anus, fistula, malrotation, colonic atresia, intussusception, and volvulus)
- neurological disorders, including Parkinson's disease, spinal cord injury, stroke, and multiple sclerosis

Any medication can come with side effects, and many have the side effect of constipation. Here are some of the most common medications which cause constipation:

- iron pills
- strong pain medications such as those containing codeine and oxycodone
- NSAIDs such as Advil, Motrin, and Aleve
- antidepressants, including tricyclic antidepressants (Elavil) and selective serotonin reuptake inhibitors (Prozac)
- psychiatric medications such as Zyprexa and Clozaril
- antacids such as Tums, which contain aluminum and calcium
- blood pressure medications including diltiazem, calcium channel blockers, beta-blockers, and nifedipine.
- allergy medications
- anti-nausea medications
- seizure and anticonvulsant medications

It's critical to remember that not everyone will have the same reaction to these medications. However, these all have been connected to an increased risk of constipation, especially with long-term use.

Risks Associated with Constipation

Anyone of any age or sex can experience constipation, and numerous factors can influence one's risk of constipation and the severity of their bout of it. These risk factors will also increase your likelihood of experiencing chronic constipation. It's important to note that there are times when you experience constipation once, and this could be for a variety of different reasons. Here are some of the factors that can increase your risk of constipation:

- **Pregnancy:** The physical and hormonal changes that someone pregnant goes through can play a large part in someone experiencing constipation. Hormonal changes make people more prone to constipation, while the physical changes cause pressure on internal organs, slowing down the movement of stool and causing constipation.
- **Diet:** Even people with the healthiest of diets can experience constipation, but a diet low in fiber is more likely to cause constipation as fiber is needed to help keep digested material moving through the GI tract.
- **Age:** Older people tend to be less active, making them more likely to experience constipation regularly. Metabolism slowing and decreased strength in muscle contraction also occur with age making it harder to have regular bowel movements.

- **Neurological and digestive issues:**
  Neurological issues affect the brain and spinal
  cord, and some of them can cause constipation
  by disrupting the communication between the
  brain and the gut.
- **Certain medications:** A side effect of many
  medications is constipation because they
  interact with our gut microbiota.

Complications Caused by Constipation

Although constipation is one of the most treated
gastrointestinal problems, many people don't seek
professional help to find the root cause of it but rather
use over-the-counter constipation medication.
However, these medications are not meant to be used
long-term, leading to health issues, especially in those
experiencing chronic constipation. Constipation,
although common, can have severe complications,
including:

- **Anal fissures:** These are tears in the lining of
  the anus which are caused by straining and
  trying to pass hardened stool.
- **Pelvic floor muscle damage:** This is also
  caused by straining, and these muscles play a
  powerful role in helping bladder control.
  Straining associated with chronic constipation

has been connected to stress urinary incontinence when urine leaks from the bladder because of too much straining.

- **Diverticulitis:** This is a condition where infections occur in the pockets that form in the intestinal wall. These pockets catch fecal matter, which can lead to infections.
- **Fecal impaction:** This is a condition that occurs when stool piles up in the rectum and anus because it is difficult to pass the stool.
- **Hemorrhoids:** This occurs when the veins around the rectum are swollen and inflamed.

CELIAC DISEASE

Celiac disease is an autoimmune gastrointestinal issue that causes the immune system to react negatively to gluten. Gluten is a group of proteins commonly found in grains, including wheat, rye, oats, and barely. Someone with Celiac disease will experience inflammation when consuming gluten. Inflammation occurs because the immune system perceives gluten as being a harmful foreign body which leads to the immune system damaging its healthy cells. Specifically, structures known as villi on the surface of the small intestine become damaged along with microvilli, both of which are essential for healthy digestion. When these become damaged, it impacts our ability to absorb nutrients, increasing our risk of malnourishment.

Celiac disease is not uncommon, with approximately 1 in 100 people worldwide having the condition and possibly not knowing it. It is estimated that about 2.5 million people in the United States alone have Celiac disease but are undiagnosed or don't know they have it (Brazier, 2017). Celiac is a life-long disease that can be treated, but the most effective way to prevent symptoms from occurring is to cut out all gluten. This disease can occur at any age.

The symptoms of Celiac disease that someone exhibits, and their severity, will differ from person to person. It also shares various symptoms with other mental and physical health conditions, which can leave people with a misdiagnosis. The age of someone with Celiac disease can also impact the symptoms someone exhibits. Children with Celiac disease can exhibit the following symptoms:

- delayed growth
- weight loss
- upset stomach
- irritability
- abdominal distention
- bloating

- recurring and chronic diarrhea
- foul-smelling, pale, and greasy stools

The symptoms of Celiac disease differ slightly in adults, and these symptoms include:

- weight loss
- gassiness
- bone and joint pain
- lack of menstruation and fertility
- irritability, depression, and mood changes
- recurring abdominal pain
- foul-smelling, pale, and greasy stools
- chronic diarrhea that is not relieved with medication
- skin rashes that are painful and itchy
- loss of enamel, tooth discoloration, and sores on the tongue and lips
- neurological problems, including headaches, poor balance, numbness and tingling in legs, seizures, and weakness

Risks Associated with Celiac Disease

Like other gastrointestinal diseases, your risk of developing Celiac disease will increase when someone genetically related to you, typically a parent or sibling has the disease. Your risk of developing Celiac disease can also increase if you already have some autoimmune disorder. This is because there are already malfunctions in the immune system, which can develop into Celiac disease. Here are the most prevalent autoimmune diseases that are associated with Celiac disease:

- anemia
- gluten ataxia
- lymphocytic colitis
- peripheral neuropathy
- type 1 diabetes
- dermatitis herpetiformis
- Down syndrome
- autoimmune thyroid disease
- chronic fatigue syndrome
- liver disease
- idiopathic dilated cardiomyopathy
- microscopic colitis
- juvenile idiopathic arthritis
- primary biliary cirrhosis
- Sjögren's syndrome

Celiac disease also comes with many health issues that can develop, especially if left untreated for a long time. You are at an increased risk of developing the following long-term health conditions if you have Celiac disease:

- heart disease
- pancreatic insufficiencies
- live failure
- lactose intolerance
- gallbladder malfunction
- early onset osteoporosis
- anemia
- infertility and miscarriage
- mineral and vitamin deficiencies
- malnutrition
- neurological conditions and symptoms, including headaches, ADHD, myopathy, ataxia, lack of muscle coordination, multifocal leukoencephalopathy, and seizures.

Triggers of Celiac Disease

Because Celiac disease revolves around gluten and the immune system's response to it, avoiding gluten is the best way to ensure you are not dealing with the symptoms. Depending on the severity of your Celiac disease, you might be able to get away with small amounts of gluten in your diet, while others might have such intolerance that even the slightest amount of gluten sets off their immune system. Here are some foods to avoid if you have Celiac disease:

- grain products, including cereals, bread, crackers, cookies, and baked goods
- soup mixes and canned soups
- processed cheese, fat-free and low-fat cottage cheese, low-fat, sour cream, and cheese mixes
- prepared and processed meats
- alcohol, including gin, whiskey, and beer
- malted barley products
- creamed vegetables
- flavored coffee
- foods with modified food starch, hydrolyzed vegetable protein, and fat substitutes and replacers

These are just a few of the many gastrointestinal diseases that can occur because of gut dysfunction. It's important to remember that these diseases are not uncommon; many millions of people experience gut health issues. Many aspects of our lives impact our gut health, and learning about these gut rivals will help you to avoid them and keep your gut happy and healthy. In the next chapter, we will learn the foods and activities you might not realize are impacting your gut health.

6

THE GUT RIVALS

There is a ton of advice in the world about what people need to do to improve their gut health, but many people ignore or overlook what they need to avoid to improve it. You can make all the good changes you want to your diet and habits, but if you are not reducing the number of negative factors, you will see little to no changes in your gut health. Reducing or completely removing things from your life that will negatively impact your gut health and overall health will allow you to see the gut health benefits you deserve. In this chapter, we will look at the biggest gut health rivals and the numerous foods, habits, activities, and medications you should avoid improving your gut health.

THE PROBLEMS WITH THE MODERN DIET

The modern diet does not promote gut health or even overall wellness. There are various issues with the modern diet, from how it is marketed to us, how peer pressure plays a part in our diets, and how it promotes obesity rather than health.

Obesity and excess weight have been the concern of health officials and people for years. Although there have been numerous health programs developed to help children and adults eat healthier and maintain a healthy weight, the rate of obesity has continued to rise. One of the reasons for this is that marketers condition their audiences to buy junk food over healthy foods. When we think about the advertisements we see for food, most of them are for junk and fast food. The ratio of healthy to unhealthy food being advertised is huge and thus unconsciously makes us buy more junk food than healthy foods because we see it more. Junk food is also marketed for cheaper, and often people can get deals such as buying in bulk or getting three for the price of two. This lures consumers into buying junk food because they perceive it as less expensive, even though they tend to buy more and spend more money in the long run.

Marketing isn't the only reason obesity and junk food are tightly linked and the problematic modern diet. Social media and peer pressure greatly influence people's buying habits. A study of 30 respondents revealed that 16 of the 30 said that social media and advertisements changed their eating habits (Thaichon & Quach, 2015). Fast food is also connected with ideals of socialization and having fun with friends, making it much harder for individuals to eat healthier regularly. During our teenage years and puberty, peer pressure is highly prevalent and plays a large part in our eating habits. Approximately 70% of teenagers will choose foods their friends prefer (Thaichon & Quach, 2015). Peer pressure can be linked not only to the place someone will eat but also to what they will eat. Look at the scenario of three friends. If two of them want to go to the same fast food place, the third one is likely to agree. If the two friends get the same meal, such as a burger with fries and a shake, there is a 75% chance that the third friend will likely get the same thing instead of choosing a healthier option (Thaichon & Quach, 2015).

It's essential to define the difference between excess weight, caused by getting unhealthy and not practicing healthy habits, and excess weight, caused by genetics. Some people are genetically inclined to be heavier, which doesn't mean they are unhealthy. They might exercise regularly and eat healthily and still have extra weight. This is very different from obesity, which is caused by a poor diet. Junk food is unhealthy because it is filled with ingredients that do not promote healthy gut microbiota and, when consumed regularly, can result in many health issues, including type 2 diabetes, heart disease, high blood pressure, cognitive decline, and even cancer. Consuming a lot of junk food is known to cause obesity because of the high amounts of sugars and fats, which cannot be used to build muscle, and thus turn into fat. These foods are also not rich in essential nutrients and vitamins that feed our gut health and don't allow our gut microbiota to flourish.

The marketing of unhealthy foods occurs from a young age, and although it might seem light, harmless advertising, it can significantly affect children's health. In 2020, it was estimated that approximately 39 million children below the age of 5 and 340 million children aged 5-19 are overweight or obese (Unicef, 2021). Marketing is partially to blame for this. Junk food is cheaper and easier, and many struggling parents will buy it over healthier alternatives. Access to junk food over healthy foods will increase the chance of someone becoming overweight. Foods that are marketed are more likely to be consumed because they are on our radar, while those not actively advertised will remain unknown to people and parents. Exposure to processed foods from a young age makes it easier to become over-weight and obese. Marketing unhealthy and ultra-processed foods have been shown to have detrimental health consequences for young children as it "creates social norms around foods and eating, increases children's preference and consumption for ultra-processed foods, and increases total energy intake" (Unicef, 2021). Poverty also plays a large part in the types of food children are exposed to, with low and middle-class families being exposed to more processed and unhealthy foods.

THE FAST-FOOD PROBLEM

Fast food has become more prominent, with fast-food chains moving into smaller and smaller towns, making them more accessible to people. It is understood that most fast-food places are not healthy, even with the healthier alternatives that many places are trying to create. The Standard American Diet (SAD) does not benefit our health but rather is detrimental. SAD has many damaging dietary factors, which can lead to numerous health concerns in the long term. These factors include:

- low in essential foods such as nuts, seeds, fruits, and vegetables
- high in trans-fats

- high in processed meats
- high in sodium
- low in omega-3 fatty acids
- low in fiber and whole grains
- high in sugar-sweetened beverages
- low in polyunsaturated fatty acids

This is the standard diet Americans consume today, but this isn't new knowledge to anyone. However, why are people still consuming this diet, knowing the risks that are associated with it? The answer to this would be that it is convenient. Going through the drive-thru after a long work day is much more convenient than going home and making a meal. Changing this mindset is essential to changing your diet and improving your gut health.

SAD is the biggest enemy of our health and can lead to numerous health issues, including diseases, disabilities, and death. Although people's life expectancy has increased thanks to technological advancements, it doesn't mean people are living in better health. They can only find better treatment for the diseases and health issues arising from their poor diets. Weight gain and obesity are the most common consequences associated with SAD; however, this diet can cause numerous health issues, including:

- **Constipation:** As we know, foods with lots of oils and fats are harder to digest, thus leading to constipation. As we discussed in the last chapter, chronic constipation can lead to many health conditions.
- **Chronic low-level inflammation:** SAD is not ideal for our gut microbiome, leading to less diversity and imbalance, which can cause chronic inflammation due to the immune system's and gut's connection.
- **Anxiety and depression:** SAD are high in saturated fats and refined carbs, which have been connected to increased levels of anxiety and depression (Stephens, n.d.). Unhealthy diets have been shown to cause a decrease in the size of the hippocampus, which is associated with memory, learning, and mood regulation. The size reduction has been linked to depression and anxiety, showing the connection between our diets and mental health.
- **Poor bone health:** SAD does not have all the essential vitamins, including vitamin K, calcium, and vitamin D, which are vital for our bone health.
- **Fatigue:** What we feed ourselves directly relates to our energy levels, as our gut turns food into

energy. Fast food and the food consumed as a part of SAD do not provide us with the right type of nourishment to keep us sustained throughout the day, leading to feelings of fatigue.

NOT GETTING ENOUGH SLEEP

Many people will put aside their sleep because they feel that they have better things to do, such as working, but sleeping is an essential thing our bodies need to do to keep our bodies and minds healthy. There is often the notion that our body and mind completely shut down when we are asleep, which is false. While we sleep, our body goes through various processes needed to ensure our overall health. Our gut health is one of the areas that need sleep to remain healthy. Studies have revealed that dysfunctions in our circadian rhythms can alter the microbiota in our intestines (Voigt et al., 2014). Our circadian rhythms are the brain's way of telling itself when to start falling asleep and when to wake. When they are functional, our brains can fall asleep and wake up at reasonable times, typically following the day and night cycles. When they are dysfunctional, our brains don't trigger sleep processes at the right time, which can make it much harder to fall asleep and stay asleep.

Sleep is essential to our gut health and vice versa. Not getting enough sleep can cause gut health issues, and gut health issues can also be the cause of sleeping problems. Healthy and diverse gut microbiomes promote good sleep. They are tightly linked, similar to our immune system and our gut. Probiotics especially have been connected to improved sleep. A study of two groups of students was conducted, with one group drinking a probiotic drink and the other drinking a placebo for eight weeks before exams. After eight weeks, the students drinking the probiotic drink reported better sleep even during a time of high stress (Laurence, 2021). However, it's important to note that different gut bacteria's effects can vary in their effectiveness from person to person. Everyone participating in the study discussed was a Japanese student. A bigger study with different ethnicities is needed to determine if the majority of people would see the same effects. The same goes for the opposite, as unhealthy gut microbiota has been linked to poor sleep.

Microbiota within our gut produces sleep-regulating hormones, including melatonin, dopamine, serotonin, and GABA (gamma-aminobutyric acid). Poor gut health will not produce enough of these hormones to help regulate sleep, resulting in inadequate sleep or the inability to fall asleep. Poor sleep is also a symptom of irritable bowel syndrome, as other symptoms, such as heartburn or abdominal pain, can make it much harder to fall asleep and stay asleep.

Effects of Poor Sleep and Sleep Deprivation

Not getting enough sleep, especially chronically, can adversely affect various areas of your life. Even after one day of poor sleep, you can see symptoms of it, including trouble focusing, feeling fatigued, and poor mood. Chronically not getting enough sleep has been linked to various health issues, including increased risk of heart disease, inflammation of the gut and other areas of the body, lowered immunity, and weight gain. While sleeping, the body goes through various processes, including repairing and boosting the immune system, further digestion, and maintaining weight. When we don't get enough sleep, our body can't do these necessary processes leading to a decline in immunity and weight gain. Weight gain occurs because our microbiomes can become imbalanced, and we can develop insulin resistance leading to weight gain and type 2 diabetes.

Sleep deprivation occurs when we are chronically not getting enough sleep and not getting good enough sleep. This means that people who might be getting the recommended amount of sleep might still experience the effects of sleep deprivation because their brain isn't able to complete the necessary cycles or get deep enough sleep to do all the things it needs. Sleep deprivation affects numerous areas of the body, including:

- **Central nervous system:** This is the main pathway of information for the body, and during sleep, nerve cells help to process information and essentially refresh the brain for the next day. When you don't get enough sleep, the brain can't refresh itself, and the next day it is already exhausted before it can start. Sleep deprivation can lead to a decline in cognitive abilities, mood swings, decreased coordination, and the development of mental and psychological issues, including impulsive behavior, depression, anxiety, paranoia, and suicidal thoughts.
- **Immune system:** Cytokines are essential infection-fighting substances in the body that are mainly produced while we are sleeping, meaning that when we are sleep deprived, our body isn't producing as defensive cells and substances, leading to a decrease in our immunity.
- **Digestive system:** Weight gain is very common in those suffering from sleep deprivation because as we sleep, the body produces leptin, a

hormone essential for telling us when we are full. Without enough sleep, the body produces more ghrelin, a hormone that triggers our appetite, and will produce less leptin, making us more prone to snacking and overeating.

- **Respiratory system:** Not getting enough sleep makes us more prone to respiratory infections, damaging our respiratory systems and making it harder to fall asleep.
- **Endocrine system:** This system is in charge of hormone production, and when we don't get enough sleep, the production of many of our hormones is disrupted. In children, especially not getting, enough sleep, their growth hormones can be affected. Growth hormones are essential for cellular and tissue repair and building muscle.
- **Cardiovascular system:** The health of our heart and blood vessels relies on sleep, and when we don't get enough sleep, it can cause an increase in inflammation, blood sugar, and blood pressure, resulting in declining cardiovascular health.

Things to Avoid to Get a Better Night Sleep

To improve your sleep, you cannot just make some positive changes, such as going to bed at the same time each night; you also need to avoid things that will compromise your ability to fall asleep and stay asleep actively. Here are some of the biggest things to avoid to ensure you get a better night's sleep:

- **Bright lights close to bedtime**: You want to expose yourself to bright light during the day, but not close to bedtime. Turn down the brightness of your phone and dim the lights in your house if possible. If you can, disconnect yourself from your phone altogether at least an hour before bed. This will help keep your circadian rhythms aligned and make it easier to fall asleep at night.

- **Consuming triggering content close to bed**: What you are consuming before bed can make it much harder to fall asleep, which is why avoiding triggering content is essential for improving your sleep. Triggering content will look different for everyone, so be sure to self-reflect and think about what triggers you and makes it harder to fall asleep.

- **Snacking too close to bedtime**: Eating too close to bedtime does not allow the body enough time to start the digestive process and can result in discomfort, heartburn, and abdominal pain while trying to fall asleep or

from waking you in the middle of the night.
You should avoid snacking one hour
before bed.

STRESSING OUT

Stress is one of the biggest threats any form of health can face. Stress occurs when our body enters into a fight or flight response because it perceives that it is in danger somehow. Most of the time, the body and mind are not in danger, but the brain perceives it is and triggers stress responses. Cortisol and adrenaline are released and are meant to help us narrow our focus and work through what is causing us stress. How people work through this problem will look very different. Those who can process their stress healthily can use it to their advantage and either complete work stressing them out or get out of a situation that is causing stress. Those unable to process their stress and cope with it appropriately tend to experience chronic stress, where health issues start to arise.

Stress can be positive, as it can help you remain motivated, but when we experience stress for too long it can negatively affect our health. Cortisol and adrenaline are not meant to be constantly produced at high levels; over time, they harm our health. Stress has been linked to various health issues, including high blood pressure, inflammation, stomach issues, a decline in cognitive abilities, anxiety, depression, and heart health issues, amongst many others.

Many things can cause stress in our lives, and they can often pile up and fester off one another, leading to one of the worst gut rivals that we can experience. What stresses something out will be different for everyone. One person might feel minimal stress in a situation, while another in the same situation might experience a much higher stress level.

Here is a list of the most common everyday activities that pile on the stress:

- **Work pressure:** There are many reasons why you might be stressed at work, including unattainable demands, lack of challenge, high penalties for mistakes, unclear requirements, and low recognition.
- **Feelings of competition:** Whether this is at work or in a hobby, feelings of competition add unneeded stress to our lives. For some people, this can be good stress, while it can add a lot of unnecessary pressure for others.
- **Rising prices of everyday items and financial responsibilities:** Financial difficulties and being financially responsible for yourself and

others comes with a lot of stress, which can be very hard to shake, especially when the cost of things continues to rise but our pay doesn't.

- **Rumination and negative thinking:** Ruminating is a form of cyclical thinking that is very difficult to break free from and increases stress. Negative thinking and a negative mindset increase stress as you focus on all the bad things that can happen rather than thinking about the positives that might come out of a situation.
- **Relationship pressure:** Being in a relationship isn't easy, because you must consider what the other person feels and what your actions mean to them. This can cause a lot of extra stress.
- **Visiting the doctor:** For some people, seeing the doctor is a big challenge because of the stress and anxiety they feel because of what they think is wrong with them.
- **Hyper-productivity:** Although this might not seem like a stressor, something that would relieve stress, hyper-productive people will often feel stressed when they don't feel productive enough.
- **Chronic list-making:** List-making is an excellent way of relieving stress and organizing your to-do list, but people who are chronic list-

makers can find it challenging to manage all the lists they are making, or they can become overwhelmed with everything they need to get done.

- **Fixing other people's problems:** Many people take on the duty of trying to fix other people's problems over their own. This puts others before themselves and adds more stress as your needs are being put on the back burner instead of being fixed. Trying to help everyone makes it very easy to become overwhelmed by everything.

- **FOMO (fear of missing out):** Being scared of missing out on something is a significant stressor, especially for young adults who see what everyone else is doing in their lives and how much they miss out on.

LEGAL POISONING

A rival to our gut health can be the medications we take to help other areas of our lives. In this situation, it is often a lose-lose situation because you will be taking medications to help with other areas of your life where you are struggling, which might be a necessary evil. Still, it is essential to try and avoid numerous medications because of their effects on our gut. However, ensuring you are not leaving other areas of your health unattended is crucial. If you need medication, take the recommended amount and try to counteract the effect you might get on your gut by making other healthy decisions that will improve your gut health. If what you are going through doesn't require medications, try different ways to improve them. For example, instead of taking an aspirin for a headache, try using aromatherapy, drinking more water, meditating, or resting your eyes. Here are some legal medications to avoid or reduce your use of for your gut health:

- **Unnecessary antibiotics:** When you don't need to be using antibiotics, avoid taking them for as much as possible. They stop the production and function of our gut's microbiota, and it can take weeks for the gut function to return to normal after taking antibiotics.
- **NSAIDs like Advil, Motrin, and Aleve:** NSAIDs are some of the most common medications; over time, they irritate the stomach, affect the gut microbiota, and cause imbalances in our gut microbiome.
- **PPIs (Proton Pump Inhibitors):** These are acid blockers commonly used to help with peptic ulcers, indigestion, and heartburn. These medications, however, also reduce the diversity

of our microbiota and increase our likelihood of infections, bone fractures, and vitamin deficiencies.

- **Antacids:** PPIs are a type of antacid, but not all antacids are PPIs. Antacids help to neutralize the acid in our stomach, but this also takes away the first line of defense that our body has against harmful pathogens. Taking antacids regularly makes us more likely to experience stomach bugs and infections.
- **Laxatives:** We use these medications because of gut health issues, but they can also affect the balance of our gut microbiome. They are not meant to be used as a long-term solution unless instructed by a doctor.

Other medications that are known to have some effect on your gut health and microbiome include sleeping pills, antidepressants, and statins. It's essential to consult with your doctor about changes in your medication or getting off of them completely, especially with medications that are helping with other conditions.

Our gut rivals are things that we can combat. Our diets are the most dangerous gut rivals, followed by not getting enough sleep, not coping with stress effectively, and the medications we are taking. The Standard

American Diet is deadly and does not promote micro-biota diversity and microbiome health. Changing our diets is essential for improving our gut health. In the next chapter, we will discuss the foods to eat to improve digestion and maintain good gut health.

7

GRABBING A QUICK, GOOD BITE

Our diets are the first area we have to look at to improve our health because what we eat feeds the microbiota in our gut. When we don't feed our microbiota the right nutrients and vitamins, we become prone to gut health issues and other health issues. In this chapter, we will explore foods that will improve your digestion, foods to limit or avoid, elimination diets, holistic and whole foods, fiber, fermented foods, food allergies vs. intolerances, and techniques to improve your digestion.

FOODS TO IMPROVE DIGESTION

The lifestyle of many people has them in a hurry to find a quick bite to eat but not paying much attention to how unhealthy the food they consume is. It's essential to change the mindset of putting eating food on the back burner. We often think that to eat healthily, we must take a long time to create extensive meals, but this isn't the case. Eating healthy is just as easy as eating unhealthy. It is vital to fuel your body with the appropriate nutrients and vitamins, and the only way to do this is to stop grabbing the quick bite to eat and grab a good bite.

Here are some of the best foods to add to your diet to help with digestion:

- **Whole grains:** Optimal gut health relies on us consuming 25 grams of fiber daily, and whole grains are the recommended grain option. Whole grains provide a lot more fiber and nutrients, aiding in producing short-chain fatty acids and promoting proper cell function.
- **Leafy greens such as kale and spinach:** These are excellent sources of fiber, folate, vitamin A, vitamin C, and vitamin K. They also contain natural sugar known for promoting the growth of healthy gut microbiota.
- **Lean protein:** Protein is essential in our diet, and the leaner it is, the easier it is to digest. People with any gut sensitivity or disorder should stick to lean proteins. Fattier proteins

trigger more intense contractions in the intestines, which can be extremely painful for those with IBD.

- **Low fructose fruits:** Reducing your overall fructose consumption can help to decrease gas and bloating, but it is also essential to have some levels of fructose. Low fructose fruits such as citrus fruits and berries not only contain fiber, but their low levels of fructose have a lower risk of causing bloating and gas.
- **Avocados:** These are considered to be a C because of the number of nutrients and fiber that are packed inside of them. They contain potassium, essential for our digestive function, and healthy fats. However, be mindful of portion sizes with avocados, as you can overeat.
- **Turmeric:** This is another superfood and is known for its anti-inflammation properties. Curcumin is a compound found in turmeric, and research has found that it can decrease inflammation, specifically in the brain (Vizthum, 2019). The anti-inflammatory properties of turmeric have been shown to help with pain and swelling associated with arthritis, which can result from chronic inflammation.
- **Ginger:** This is one of the best-known foods for helping with nausea, diarrhea, and upset

stomach. It is available in numerous forms and, when eaten regularly, can help with chronic stomach pain.

- **Omega-3 fatty acids:** These are found in chia, fish, walnuts, flax, hemp, and algae. Omega-3 fatty acids are essential for a healthy gut microbiome and overall health, as they help structure our cells and keep our immune system healthy.
- **Whole food fats:** These are found in olives, nuts, seeds, and avocados. We often think that we need to cut out fats entirely, but there are different types of fat. Whole food fats are the most beneficial, but you must ensure you don't eat too many fats.

FOODS TO LIMIT AND AVOID

Now that you know the foods to start including in your diet more, it's time to learn about the foods you should limit or avoid. I'm not saying to cut out these foods because when consumed moderately entirely and with a balanced diet, they won't have the adverse effects they have when overconsumed. It's important to enjoy your food sometimes, which sometimes means eating junk food. Here is a list of food to limit how much you eat or avoid:

- **High-intensity sweeteners used as sugar alternatives:** As we have learned, sweeteners, although they are an alternative to sugar, are not healthy, and they can be harmful to our gut health and even contain harmful bacteria for our gut health.

- **Milk or lactose-based foods:** Lactose-intolerance is very common, and when someone has this condition or is sensitive toward milk to other dairy products, they can experience gas, bloating, abdominal pain, and diarrhea when consuming food or drinks with lactose. Avoiding these foods when lactose intolerant can significantly improve your gut health.

- **Foods high in fructose/fruit sugar:** Processed foods, soft drinks, and sweets contain high amounts of high fructose corn syrup which can aggravate symptoms of IBS or other gut health issues. Large consumption of high fructose corn syrup has been linked to an increased risk of insulin resistance and the development of type 2 diabetes. Avoid fruits high in fructose and opt for those low in it, such as berries and citrus fruit.

- **Carbonated beverages:** Did you know the fizziness in carbonated drinks does not stop once we drink them? It continues with this effect throughout the GI tract, which can cause irritation, bloating, and abdominal pain. Carbonated drinks such as soda are also high in fructose corn syrup.

- **Caffeine:** Coffee is one of the most common forms of caffeine and one of the most popular beverages out there, but caffeine has been shown to aggravate symptoms of IBS, such as diarrhea, and it can increase anxiety.

ELIMINATION DIETS

Elimination diets sound a lot more intense than they are. In this diet, you are going to create a meal plan for yourself, or with the aid of professionals, which will have you avoiding ingredients and foods that you suspect or know that you have an intolerance, sensitivity, or allergy to. Elimination diets are not about losing weight or improving your overall diet. They are more about learning what might be causing you any gut health issues or exacerbating symptoms of diseases.

Once you have identified possible foods or ingredients you are intolerant or sensitive to, you need to eliminate them from your diet completely. You should do this for about two or three weeks. The elimination phase should help you to determine if the foods you have cut out are the ones causing your symptoms. After you have cut them out for two or three weeks, it is time to start slowly introducing them back into your diet. You must be very slow in your reintroduction so as not to become confused by which food is causing symptoms. Try introducing one of the eliminated foods each week and be diligent in examining yourself and being mindful of any symptoms.

You want to be as strict as possible for the best outcome from this diet. Here is a list of the common foods that people will cut out during their elimination diet:

- legumes: lentils, beans, soy-based products, and peas
- citrus fruits: grapefruits and oranges
- nuts and seeds
- meat and fish: processed meats, chicken, pork, beef, cold cuts, shellfish, and eggs
- nightshade vegetables: peppers, eggplants, tomatoes, cayenne peppers, paprika, and potatoes
- dairy products: milk, cheese, yogurt, and ice cream
- starches: barley, corn, wheat, oats, bread, rye, and spelt
- fats: margarine, hydrogenated oils, spreads, butter, mayonnaise

- sugar and sweets: sugar, maple syrup, corn syrup, honey, agave nectar, desserts, high fructose corn syrup, and chocolate

HOLISTIC AND WHOLE FOODS

Holistic and whole foods are essentially real food. They are foods that are in their natural state and are free of chemical additives, unprocessed, and high in nutrients. Processed foods were a modern invention, being created in the 20th century. They emerged with the creation of the Western diet and served as ready-to-eat meals. Processed foods rose to popularity because of their convenience, but before the modern era, all that was available were whole foods —and people were arguably much healthier. Holistic and whole foods allow you to get the most nutrients from your diet and maintain your gut and overall health.

Here are six reasons to eat whole foods:

1. **Loaded in nutrients:** Processed foods are unhealthy because they lack sufficient nutrients and contain chemicals and additives. Whole foods don't contain any additives and are choke full of nutrients. It takes a lot less consumption of whole foods to reach the daily recommended

amount of nutrients than it does with processed foods.

2. **High in fiber:** As we know, fiber is essential for our diets because it boosts our gut function, feelings of fullness, and metabolic health. People commonly take fiber supplements but getting it from whole foods is always recommended as the effects will last longer.

3. **Low in sugar:** Sugary foods are linked to an increased risk of insulin resistance, type 2 diabetes, obesity, and heart disease, amongst others. Processed foods are usually full of sugar, while whole foods contain a lot less sugar when sugar is present.

4. **Reduce disease risk:** When we eat processed foods, our risk of developing numerous diseases increases. Switching to a diet of whole foods can significantly decrease your risk of disease, including heart disease and cancer.

5. **Good for your gut:** What you put into your gut affects its health, and processed foods are the worst. Whole foods are great for our gut microbiomes and feed the microbiota that lives in our gut. Many whole foods also serve as prebiotics which is essential for gut health.

6. **Provides variety:** Many processed foods are very similar to one another and don't provide

the variety our diets need to promote a diverse microbiome. Thousands of whole foods out there can give you so much variety.

FIBER

Fiber is essential to our gut health. Whether incorporating it by taking supplements or eating more food high in fiber, getting more fiber in your diet is an essential step to improving your gut health. Fiber is integral in how our digestive tract functions, including digesting food and maintenance. Two kinds of fiber can be consumed: soluble and insoluble. Soluble fiber dissolves in water and is digestible by the good bacteria in our gut. Insoluble fiber does not dissolve. Another way to categorize it is as fermentable and non-fermentable. Most foods contain a combination of both soluble and insoluble fiber. Here are the ways that fiber is essential for your gut health:

- **Feeds good bacteria:** Most of the body's bacteria live within the intestines, which is why eating foods that feed your good gut bacteria is essential. The intestines contain enzymes that break down fiber and feed the bacteria in the intestine. The production of good bacteria then helps to decrease our likelihood of developing disorders such as Crohn's, IBS, and ulcerative colitis.

- **Can help you lose weight:** Only some types of fiber can do this, and they do it by making us feel fuller faster and thus reducing how much we eat.
- **Keeps the lining of the gut intact:** Our gut is essential, and when it's not intact, it can lead to various health issues, including ulcerative colitis. The gut lining serves as a protector because it allows water and certain bacteria to enter and keeps harmful bacteria and pathogens out.
- **Keeps gut microbiota balanced:** Balance in the gut microbiome is essential for our health. When there is an imbalance, it leads to numerous health issues. Fiber keeps the production of good microbiota up and promotes diversity, thus keeping everything balanced. Fiber helps the function of all good microbiota.

FERMENTED FOODS

The word fermented might not seem all that appetizing, but many foods are fermented and have numerous benefits for our gut health. Some examples of fermented foods include kimchi, pickles, and sauerkraut. The fermentation process is used to make products last longer, but it also boosts the nutritional value of the food as it increases the probiotics in the food. Probiotics are living microorganisms found in some foods and are incredibly beneficial for our gut health. Fermented foods are a great item to add to your diet, and if you are still questioning this, here are some of the benefits of consuming fermented foods:

- **Helps with digestion:** Fermented foods and their living microorganisms help break down food as they boost good microbiota and digestion.
- **Helps fight harmful bacteria:** Harmful bacteria and pathogens are constantly at war with our good microbiota. Eating fermented foods will help boost the healthy microbiota and fight off illness and infection. Fermented foods lower the pH levels in our intestines, reducing the production of harmful bacteria.
- **Can restore gut health after using antibiotics:** As we know, antibiotics are highly harmful to our gut health, and it can take months to get our gut microbiome back to normal functioning. Eating fermented foods helps to restore gut health.

- **Helps produce vitamins:** Vitamins are essential for the body, and fermented foods help produce many vitamins, including vitamin K and vitamins B1, B2, B3, B6, and B12.
- **Creates balance within the gut:** Fermented foods help to boost the diversity in our gut and keep it balanced.

FOOD ALLERGIES AND SENSITIVITIES VS. FOOD INTOLERANCES

Food allergies occur when the immune system deems certain ingredients or food as being a danger and triggers numerous effects that can be life-threatening, including rashes, hives, and swelling. Anaphylaxis occurs when the immune system's reaction to a trigger is extreme and can be life-threatening. The severity of someone's allergy can differ.

Food sensitivities can often be compared to less severe versions of allergies as they create a reaction but are frequently delayed. The reactions the immune system has to these foods are very rarely life-threatening. The symptoms associated with someone's food sensitivity can take days to show up, which can sometimes make it hard to pinpoint just what is causing the symptoms someone is experiencing. Because the reactions can be so delayed and minute, people can go their entire lives

152 | OLIVIA SIMON

without knowing they have food sensitivity. Signs of food sensitivity include migraines, diarrhea, and bloating.

Unlike food allergies and sensitivity, intolerances to certain foods are not caused by the immune system, but rather because your digestive system has a hard time breaking down certain foods—often because it lacks an enzyme to do so. The symptoms of food intolerance include bloating, upset stomach, and diarrhea, but they are not life-threatening. These symptoms typically occur shortly after eating and as your body starts to digest the food. Depending on the severity of someone's intolerance, eating a small amount of a trigger food might not cause a reaction.

TECHNIQUES TO IMPROVE DIGESTION

Improving your digestion first starts with improving the food that you eat. We know that our microbiota influences our gut functions and that certain foods will hinder or help the functions of our microbiota. Eating healthier is not the only way to improve your digestion. There are multiple different techniques that one can use to improve their diet. Try these techniques to improve your digestion:

- **Exercise:** Getting up and moving is a great way to keep your digestion healthy. A part of digestion is your food moving downward through the body. Moving around allows gravity to help keep the food moving and make digestion easier and faster. Bloating can also be reduced by walking as it keeps food moving throughout the digestive system. Exercise also increases blood flow to muscles, making it easier for our digestive system to move food.
- **Avoid triggering foods:** A part of improving digestion is being sure to avoid triggering foods. If you know a food is going to cause you digestive issues, avoid it. This will reduce digestive symptoms and improve your overall digestion as it won't need to work harder to digest triggering foods.
- **Keep a food diary:** You might not always be aware of the foods that trigger you, or maybe you want to diversify your diet more; either way, keeping a food diary can help. You can track the types of foods you are eating and if you have any symptoms. You can also use it to prep meals for the week or write down ideas for different recipes you want to try.
- **Stay hydrated:** Hydration is essential for our digestive health. Fluids help to keep food and

waste products moving throughout the
digestive system.

Now that you know which foods to eat more of and
which to avoid, you can start exploring foods to add to
your diet or which to remove. In the next chapter, we
will discuss diet etiquette and a sample meal plan that
women can try to improve their gut health.

8

WHAT HEALTHY EATING LOOKS LIKE

Did you know that 70% of Americans report their diet is healthy despite the massive amounts of evidence that says the opposite (Aubrey & Godoy, 2016)? Some of the evidence that contradicts these statements includes that nearly 80% of Americans don't eat the recommended servings of fruits or vegetables and that 36% of American adults are classified as obese (Aubrey & Godoy, 2016). It's important to note that diet isn't the only factor that dictates someone's weight, but it plays a big part. The poor diet that most Americans have links back to nearly 40% of Americans experiencing some form of gut health issues (Aubrey & Godoy, 2016), showing that our nutrition is key to our gut health. This chapter will look at dieting etiquette and a sample meal plan for women to improve their gut health.

FREQUENTLY ASKED QUESTIONS ABOUT A GUT-FRIENDLY DIET

Starting one might seem nearly impossible without knowing what a gut-friendly diet is. We've learned all about what makes a gut-friendly diet, but there are still many questions you might have about gut-friendly diets and how to maintain them. Here are some of the most frequently asked questions about gut-friendly diets:

- **How common are gut issues?**

  As we know, gut health issues are very common, and women are more prevalent to experience them than men. In Western society, gut health issues are more prominent because of the increased use of antibiotics, eating nutrient-poor foods regularly, and high alcohol consumption, all of which poorly affect our gut microbiota and lead to gut health issues.

- **What does a gut-friendly diet look like?**

A gut-friendly diet will cut out harmful foods to your gut health, remove triggering foods, and incorporate healthy foods and good eating habits into your diet.

- **How can you tell if your gut is improving?**

How quickly your gut improves and how much difference you notice will be different for everyone. One of the first improvements that people see is a reduction in heartburn. However, you won't see this improvement if you don't have a lot of heartburn. Other symptoms that someone will see a decrease in include bloating, cramping, and abdominal pain. When sticking to a meal plan, people can also see weight loss. Other improvements one might see in life include better mood and clearer skin.

- **Are gut diet plans challenging and restrictive?**

There is often the stigma that diets are restrictive, but gut-friendly diets are the opposite, with many people surprised by the variety and flavor of foods they get to eat. Gut-health diets provide variety, and it's important to remember that not all calories are equal. Chicken is a common protein used in gut-friendly diets because it's rich in nutrients and takes a while to digest, which burns more calories. It's essential to remain organized during a gut-friendly diet.

- **How do I maintain good gut health?**

Maintaining your good gut health is all up to you. You must be willing to make the changes to your diet and maintain them to keep your gut health good. A part of good gut health is changing your mindset and habits about food and eating. Keeping your old habits and mindset will make it hard to maintain good gut health.

LOW FODMAP DIET

A Low FODMAP diet is one of the best gut-friendly diets that people looking to improve their gut health can adopt. This diet removes short-chain carbohydrates (FODMAP) that the gut can't absorb properly, leading to multiple gut symptoms. FODMAP stands for "fermentable oligosaccharides, disaccharides, monosaccharides, and polyols" (Migala, 2021). This diet focuses on eliminating foods from your diet that might cause digestive issues, including constipation, bloating, gas, cramping, and diarrhea. This diet will remove possible triggering foods before adding them back into your diet. If this sounds similar, this diet is very similar to the elimination diets we discussed in a previous chapter. You will want to avoid certain foods for four weeks, and then after the four weeks, you can start reintroducing the foods back into your diet. The reintroduction of high FODMAP foods will show you which ones are causing your digestive issues, and you can avoid them.

Foods you can eat on a Low FODMAP diet include bell pepper, Bok choy, banana, brie cheese, carrots, cucumbers, dark chocolate, eggplant, eggs, feta cheese, firm tofu, fish and seafood, green beans, grapes, hard cheeses, kiwi, orange, oatmeal, oats, olives, peanuts, peanut butter, popcorn, plain non-marinated meats, pineapple, potatoes, sourdough bread, strawberries, and tomatoes.

Foods to avoid while on a Low FODMAP diet include asparagus, artichoke, apples, beans, barley, blackberries, cauliflower, cow's milk, cherries, cashews, garlic, honey, lentils, mango, nectarines, pasta, pears, pistachios, rye, soy milk, watermelon, wheat, and yogurt.

Foods that can be eaten but should be moderated include avocado (1/8 portion), broccoli (3/4 cup), cabbage (3/4 cup), canned pumpkin (1/3 cup), and sweet potato (1/2 cup).

Anyone can try the Low FODMAP diet, but it is highly recommended for people with IBS, and it has been shown to reduce symptoms in almost 86% of people who try the diet (Veloso, n.d.), making it one of the most successful treatments and diets for people with IBS or other gut health issues.

Underweight people, who have a history of eating disorders, or have poor eating habits should avoid Low FODMAP diets as they can seem too restricting or not provide adequate nourishment, especially if you are already malnourished. Most foods containing FODMAP are healthy; it's just a matter of finding out which ones might exacerbate any digestive symptoms you are experiencing.

GETTING INTO SHAPE

A part of going on a diet is improving your gut health, but you might also want to get into better shape. A part of getting into shape is not only about exercising and eating the right foods; it's about creating the perfect space for you when it comes to cooking and living a gut-friendly life. Here are some tips for creating the ideal gut-friendly space for you:

- **Create a dedicated space for gut-friendly food:** Removing the temptation of unhealthy foods and having a space for gut-friendly food can significantly improve your health.
- **Gather essentials ahead of time:** Make a list and gather food ahead of time. Stick to the list to avoid buying unnecessary foods.
- **Claim YOUR kitchen counter!** Have your own space that no one else uses. Fewer people in the kitchen mean you have more control over what you eat.
- **Involve your friends/family in your journey:** Call on them to motivate you and keep you accountable.
- **Use your refrigerator door to inspire you:** Print off recipes or inspirational quotes and stick them to the fridge to motivate you to try new things and stick to your diet.
- **Shrink your plate:** When you have a large plate, you often feel the need to fill it up completely, leading to overeating and digestive problems. Shrinking your plate size can reduce how much you are eating, allowing your gut to not be overloaded.

- **Don't eat in front of the TV:** Eating in front of the TV takes your attention away from the food, and can lead to overeating.
- **Store spices and your specific items in fun baskets:** Making the kitchen fun will make you want to spend time in it. Having spices on hand also allows you to customize meals.
- **Keep the kitchen clean:** A messy kitchen is not one people want to spend time in. Keeping it clean makes cooking more fun and enjoyable.
- **Know what you'll be eating tomorrow:** Create a meal plan a day or week ahead so that you are not standing in the kitchen, debating on what you will cook, and just grabbing an unhealthy snack because you can't decide.
- **Be open to hiring or recruiting help to gather and cook meals.**

MEALS TO TRY

It is time to cut out harmful foods from your diet and add positive foods and experiences instead. Making your meals, enjoying them, and knowing they are healthy is an amazing experience and can be an excellent motivator for improving your gut health. Here is a sample of the daily meal plan you can create to help your gut health. These include just one recipe for each meal, but there is an infinite number of meals you can try.

Breakfast: Overnight Oats

Ingredients (yields four servings):

- 2 cups of milk (dairy or unsweetened non-dairy milk)
- 2 cups of old-fashioned rolled oats
- 1 cup of yogurt (Greek or non-dairy)
- 3 tablespoons of honey or maple syrup
- 1/4 teaspoon of kosher salt
- 1/4 teaspoon of cinnamon
- optional: 1 tablespoon of chia seeds
- optional toppings: nuts, nut butter, fruits, or seeds

Instructions:

1. Combine all ingredients in a large bowl.
2. Divide combined ingredients into individual containers.
3. Put in the refrigerator for at least 4 hours, but preferably overnight.
4. Stir the mixture before eating and top with desired ingredients.
5. Store overnight oats for up to 4 days.

Nutritional Information: 291 calories, 11.6 grams of protein, 47.9 grams of carbs, 4.6 grams of fiber, 6.9 grams of fat, and 17.3 grams of sugar.

Lunch: Grilled Chicken Thighs, Shrimp, or Salmon with Pineapple Mint Salsa

Ingredients (yields six servings):

Chicken:

- 3 pounds of skin-on, bone-in chicken thighs (can be substituted with different proteins such as shrimp or salmon)
- 1/2 teaspoon of garlic powder
- 1/2 teaspoon of ginger powder
- 1/2 teaspoon of sea salt

Salsa:

- 1/2 of a large pineapple, cut into half-inch chunks
- 1 cucumber, cut into half-inch chunks
- 1 bunch of radishes, cut into half-inch chunks and tops cut off
- 1 avocado, cut into half-inch chunks
- 1 bunch of green onions, tops, and roots removed, finely chopped
- 1 clove of garlic, minced

- 1 ounce of finely chopped mint leaves
- juice from half a lemon
- 1/2 teaspoon of ginger powder
- 1/2 teaspoon of sea salt

Instructions:

1. Combine spices and salt in a bowl.
2. Rinse and dry the chicken. Rub the spice mix into the chicken until coated.
3. Heat grill and add chicken, skin-side down when it is hot.
4. Cook for 5-7 minutes or until skin is crispy and flip. Cook for another 5-7 minutes. If you have a thermometer, the internal heat of the chicken should be 165 degrees Fahrenheit.
5. Combine salsa ingredients into a bowl and stop chicken with salsa.

Nutritional Information: 529 calories, 33 grams of protein, 16 grams of carbs, 4 grams of fiber, 37 grams of fat, 9 grams of saturated fat, and 9 grams of sugar.

Dinner: Creamy Vegan Garlic Pasta with Roasted Tomatoes

Ingredients (yields four servings):

- 10 ounces of whole-wheat pasta
- 3 cups of grape or cherry tomatoes, cut into halves
- 2 1/2 cups of unsweetened, plain Almond Breeze
- 8 garlic cloves, grated or minced
- 2 medium shallots, diced
- 3-4 tablespoons of all-purpose flour
- 2-3 tablespoons of nutritional yeast
- sea salt and pepper
- olive oil
- optional: 1-2 tablespoons of lemon juice
- optional: 1-2 tablespoons of parmesan cheese, preferably vegan

Instructions:

1. Preheat oven to 400 degrees Fahrenheit and prepare a baking sheet with parchment paper.
2. Toss tomatoes with olive oil and salt, and place, cut side down on the prepared baking sheet.
3. Bake for 20 minutes.

4. Prepare pasta according to package, drain, cover, and let sit.

5. Place a large skillet over medium-low heat and add one tablespoon of olive oil, shallot, garlic, salt, and pepper. Stir frequently for 3-4 minutes.

6. Add flour to skillet and stir with a whisk. Once combined, whisk in almond milk and nutritional yeast. Keep whisking to make sure there are no clumps. Add more salt and pepper and allow to simmer. Cook for 4-5 minutes.

7. For a creamier sauce, blend until smooth. Taste and adjust the seasoning as you like.

8. Add tomatoes and pasta to the sauce once prepared as your life.

9. Add lemon and parmesan cheese if you desire.

Nutritional Information: 379 calories, 11.5 grams of protein, 64 grams of carbs, 8.5 grams of fiber, 0.8 grams of saturated fat, and 5 grams of sugar.

Trying new foods and creating meal plans is a great way to improve your gut health, but sometimes this can be very hard for some people. Fiber and other nutrients are essential for our gut health, and if you don't think your diet is giving you enough, gut supplements might be the best option for you; in the next chapter, we will learn all about them.

9

THE GUT SUPPLEMENTS

We have to have more than fiber to keep our gut healthy. Ensuring that your diet has lots of variety and that you are taking supplements for the areas that you are lacking or when you need a boost will help to keep your gut at optimal health. Nutrients and supplements are necessary for our gut health, and in this chapter, we will explore the importance of prebiotics, probiotics, postbiotics, and phytochemicals.

PREBIOTICS, PROBIOTICS, AND POSTBIOTICS —AN OVERVIEW

Throughout this book, we have discussed the importance of prebiotics, their importance, and why you need to incorporate them into your diet more. But let's recap what a probiotic is. Probiotics are "live microorganisms that, when administered in adequate amounts, confer a health benefit on the host" (Hill et al., 2014). Probiotics are essentially living microorganisms that contain beneficial bacteria that provide numerous gut benefits.

Probiotics are created through fermentation and can be found in many foods. Common examples of fermented foods include kimchi, sauerkraut, yogurt, kefir, kombucha tea, unpasteurized pickles, and pickled vegetables.

Probiotics can also be taken as a supplement, especially if you aren't the fondest of the taste of fermented foods or find it harder to get them into your diet regularly. However, probiotics from food can be much more effective because they also have fiber which our gut microbiota can feed on.

Prebiotics and Dietary Fiber

People often think they need to take prebiotic supplements, but this isn't the case. Prebiotics are found in carbs, mostly fiber, and cannot be digested by the human body. However, they are essential for our gut health as they feed our gut microbiota. Many of the foods that we eat contain prebiotics, including legumes, berries, bananas, oats, peas, beans, dandelion greens, garlic, leeks, onions, asparagus, and Jerusalem arti-chokes. Prebiotic fiber is turned into short-chain fatty acids, such as butyrate. The body can't produce enough butyrate without adequate prebiotics in our diets. The microbiota ferments short-chain fatty acids in our intestines, and they stimulate the production of beneficial bacteria.

Examples of prebiotics include:

- FOS (fructo- oligosaccharide)
- GOS (galacto-oligosaccharides)
- polyols (sugar alcohols) used as nutritive sweeteners

Postbiotics

Postbiotics are the byproducts of our gut microbiota fermenting probiotics. A cycle occurs in our guts, which is as follows: Probiotics are fed by prebiotics, which then is fermented and creates postbiotics. Although they are technically a waste product, they have lots of health-boosting properties, including:

- **Prevent obesity and lower blood pressure:** increase the amount of gut microbiota we have in our gut, which can help lower blood pressure and prevent insulin resistance and obesity.

- **Support probiotics:** probiotics and postbiotics work together, and we need postbiotics to support the immunomodulatory effects which support probiotics and their functions.
- **Antimicrobial properties:** our gut is an ecosystem, and it needs bacteria-fighting properties to promote healthy microbiota growth; postbiotics have antimicrobial properties that keep the ecosystem clean and healthy.
- **Treats diarrhea:** they interact with the good bacteria of our intestinal walls and help to treat diarrhea.
- **Reduces inflammation:** postbiotics help to boost beneficial microbiota, which helps to reduce inflammation, specifically in the intestines.
- **Support immune system functions:** infants and those immunocompromised will see this effect much more than others, as postbiotic compounds will be safer to use than probiotics because they are much more tolerable for the gut.

Postbiotics are harder to come by and are often not labeled as postbiotics. Rather when looking online or in stores, look for labels such as dried yeast fermentate, sodium butyrate, and calcium butyrate. Because postbiotics are created through fermentation in our gut microbiome, eating more prebiotics and probiotics.

PHYTOCHEMICALS

Phytochemicals are compounds found in plants and give plants their flavor, color, and aroma. There are thousands of phytochemicals, and they play different roles within the plants and when we eat them. However, knowledge of the many roles of phytochemicals is still being explored. Preliminary studies reveal that people who eat a primarily plant-based diet are less likely to develop diseases and cancer, which is thought to be caused by phytochemicals (Roswell Park Comprehensive Cancer Center, 2019).

There are thousands of types of phytochemicals, but we only know a few of them and their potential benefits. Here are a few that we know of:

- **Carotenoids:** inhibit cancer cell growth, boost immunity, and reduce the risk of heart disease. Found in cooked carrots, sweet potatoes, orange squash, tomatoes, and green plants, including broccoli.
- **Flavonoids:** fight inflammation, reduce tumor growth, and decrease DNA damage. Found in

walnuts, soybeans, apples, berries, tea, citrus
fruits, whole grains, and coffee.

- **Anthocyanins:** help lower blood pressure and
  are found in berries.
- **Isothiocyanates:** can help protect against heart
  disease and cancer. Found in cruciferous
  vegetables, including kale, broccoli, and
  cauliflower.
- **Lutein and zeaxanthin:** can promote eye
  health and are found in dark leafy greens like
  chard and spinach.

Why Are They Essential for Health?

Phytochemicals have so many benefits, as you can see
from the list of types that we have listed. One type of
phytochemical essential to our health is antioxidants,
which help reduce oxidative stress or the byproduct of
our body and brain doing necessary processes. When
we don't have enough antioxidants, we can experience
negative symptoms of too much oxidative stress,
including inflammation. Depending on the phytochemical, there will be different benefits, but here are the
known benefits:

- help regulate your emotions
- reduce inflammation
- aid immune system functions

- slow cancer cell growth
- protect DNA and cells from damage

Fruits and vegetables are essential for our diets because of the wide range of benefits we get from phytochemicals. Although we are supposed to eat fruits and vegetables regularly, many people struggle to include them in their diets. Here are some easy ways to incorporate phytochemicals into your diet:

- Instead of eating candies, opt for dried fruits such as pineapples, apricots, apples, or a mix of tropical fruits.
- Add vegetables such as onions, spinach, artichokes, or sliced tomatoes to your pizza.
- Add grated apples, carrots, or zucchini to the muffin mix.
- Speed up meal prep with jars of chopped basil, ginger, or garlic.
- Use ketchup instead of mayonnaise.
- Make an effort to eat five portions of fruits and vegetables a day.
- Eat the albedo, or white parts, of citrus fruits.
- Eat fruits instead of drinking fruit juice.
- Cook with whole grains, including whole oats, quinoa, brown rice, barley, buckwheat, and amaranth.

- Try soy products like vegetable protein meat and tofu.

Think about what you are missing from your diet. Although it's been missing until now, you can start to change that today. You can change your diet today by adding more healthy foods that provide prebiotics, probiotics, and phytochemicals, all of which can help improve your diet and gut health. Don't worry about failing; just think about how you will start again. After improving your diet, it's time to make some habit changes. In the next chapter, we will discuss exercising and your gut health.

10

EXERCISING FOR GUT HEALTH

The research behind the benefits of exercising on one's gut health and overall health is astronomical. Research has found that exercising regularly for six weeks can help restore your gut's natural functions (Pratt, 2018). Depending on your gut health issues, how much function is regained will differ. People with gut health diseases will see less improvement. In this chapter, we will discuss different exercises to do to improve your health.

EXERCISING AND GUT HEALTH

Exercising is essential for your gut and overall health. Too many high-intensity workouts can cause gut health issues, but a well-rounded exercise routine and regular physical activity can benefit your gut health. Different exercises have different effects on gut health. One of the most significant benefits of exercising on gut health is increased blood flow to the digestive system and allowing digestive material to move. Working out your abdominals also makes your intestines move, which aids in digestion.

The gut microbiome is also changed when someone is getting regular exercise. A study revealed that people who exercised for 30-60 minutes three times a week saw positive changes in their gut microbiota (Pratt, 2018). The changes that can occur to our gut microbiome because of exercising are caused by microbiome sensitivity. Microbiome sensitivity refers to changes in our gut microbiota because of changes in circulating hormones, blood flow, and intensity motility.

Lifestyle plays a large part in your gut health. You might be getting regular exercise, but if you aren't practicing other healthy habits, you might not see as much of an improvement in your gut health as you would like. People who are under a lot of stress, don't eat healthily, don't get enough sleep, or practice other unhealthy habits, can still have gut health issues even when exercising regularly.

Here are some of the most powerful exercises you can use to improve your gut health:

- **Yoga:** Various yoga positions have been tied to improved gut health, including cat-cow stretch, standing forward bend, camel pose, triangle pose, and thunderbolt/diamond pose.
- **Walking:** Do a daily walkie/talkie, and use the time to catch up with family or friends,
- **Walking meditation and walking with intention:** These forms of walking have a purpose and an intention of improving your gut health. Walking meditation has you reflecting on what you feel as you meditate.
- **Biking:** This exercise helps the movement of digestive material through the digestive system. It helps reduce water loss in stools which improve digestion.
- **Sit-ups or crunches:** These get your abdominal muscles moving, which gets your digestive system moving. They help with bloating and gas as well.
- **Pelvic floor activation:** To do this, squeeze and draw in the muscles of the anus and vagina. This should feel like you are lifting them. Breathe slowly in and out. Over time, this exercise can help with bowel movements and bladder control.
- **Breathing exercise:** Diaphragmatic breathing can be highly beneficial for gut health as it helps

you cope with stress, which causes less strain on the gut. Deep breathing before eating can also help with digestion.

Workouts for Gut Health

Different exercises target different areas of the body, and they can have different effects on your gut health. Here are different workouts you can use to improve your gut health.

Abs Blaster

This exercise is a great one to try if you are feeling constipated. This exercise is excellent for those that suffer from constipation because of the rhythmic ab movement, which helps to encourage bowel movement and increase blood flow. To do this exercise, you will do ten different ab exercises in 10 minutes.

- Duration: 10 minutes
- Intensity: high
- Equipment needed: none
- Suitable for: intermediate or advanced

Gut-Boost

This gut-boosting exercise is a full-body exercise that works out deep core muscles, obliques, and abdominals. Combining this exercise with the HIIT method is a great way to burn calories, get your heart rate pumping, and increase blood flow.

- Duration: 12 minutes
- Intensity: moderate to intense
- Equipment needed: none
- Suitable for: everyone

For this workout, you will do the following exercises:

1. High knees running in place for 30 seconds. You can make this low impact by doing it at a slower speed.
2. Bicycle crunches for 30 seconds
3. Mountain climbers for 30 seconds
4. Burpees for 30 seconds
5. Repeat these exercises three or four times and rest for one minute in between each exercise

Cardio Ab Workout

Exercising your abs will always help with digestion as you activate your abdominal muscles, which can help move digested food through the intestines. The mix of cardio and ab workouts is a great way to get your blood flowing and heart pumping. For this movement, you will do both cardio and ab workouts for 30 minutes.

- Duration: 30 minutes
- Intensity: high
- Equipment needed: exercise mat
- Suitable for: everyone

Mat Flow Workout

Yoga is an excellent exercise for beginners as it is short, relaxing, and gentle. You can practice yoga anywhere, and it doesn't require going to the gym or having any materials except a yoga mat. The Mat Flow workout uses therapeutic posture, twists, and breathwork to stimulate the digestive system. Yoga can also help to reset and detoxify. Mat Flow is essentially any form of yoga aimed at digestion.

- Duration: 18 minutes
- Intensity: low
- Equipment needed: yoga mat
- Suitable for: everyone

Tips for Optimizing Your Workout

People often think that working out takes a long time and that they don't have enough time to incorporate it into their routine. However, this isn't the case. The exercises we just discussed are all short; what matters is not how long you work out but how much you optimize your workout to best fit your schedule. When it comes to your gut health, there are multiple ways you can optimize your workout to allow for more improvements in your gut health. Here are some tips for optimizing your workout to improve your gut health:

- **Opt for a low-intensity and low-impact workout:** You don't always need to be going super hard or fast when working out. This is a bad thing because it can lead to you becoming injured. High-intensity workouts can be very hard on the gut because blood flow is not increased to the gut but rather goes to the muscles as they are under the most strain. The decreased blood flow causes the digestive system to slow. Opting for low-intensity and low-impact workouts gives you the benefits of exercising without the strain on your digestive system.
- **Don't skip HIIT (high-intensity interval training):** Although high-impact and high-intensity workouts can cause adverse effects when done constantly, it's important not to skip HIIT. Inflammation can occur when someone does too much HIIT, but taking a high-quality probiotic can counteract this.

- **Bring mindfulness to your workout:** Working out without a goal in mind or intention can make it very hard to become motivated and stick with a workout plan. Be mindful of the exercises you choose and the outcome you want from them because it makes it much easier to be motivated and stick with your plan.

7-Day Workout Plan

Try this 7-day workout plan to get started on incorporating exercise into your routine and improving your gut health:

Day 1:

- Morning: yoga
- Evening: ab blaster

Day 2:

- Morning: sit-ups
- Evening: walking meditation

Day 3:

- Morning: cardio ab workout
- Evening: breathing exercises

Day 4:

- Morning: biking
- Evening: Yoga

Day 5:

- Morning: walking with intention
- Evening: mat flow workout

Day 6:

- Morning: sit-ups
- Evening: Walking

Day 7:

- Morning: gut-boosting exercise
- Evening: pelvic floor activation

Physical exercise is essential for gut and overall health. You now know which exercises are best for your gut health. Your gut health isn't only affected by what you eat. Your brain and mental health play a large part in your gut health, and in the next chapter, we will discuss the correlation between brain health and gut health.

11

BRAIN HEALTH = GUT HEALTH

We have to look at our overall health to see an improvement in our gut health. As we learned earlier in this book, there is a profound connection between our gut and brain. When one is under duress, we can often see symptoms in the other. Remember that our gut health is not restricted to what we eat. Practicing healthy habits in all areas of life is essential for gut health. Throughout this chapter, we will talk about meditation and its benefits, tips for improving sleep, and methods for reducing stress. It might seem very hard at first to make the right changes to your life, such as getting enough sleep and reducing stress, but I have been at the starting point as you are now, and the benefits are worth it in the end.

MEDITATION

Meditation has been practiced for thousands of years in various cultures worldwide. Depending on the culture, the purpose behind meditation might change, but everyone who uses it can get the immense amounts of benefits that it has on our mental and physical health. How meditation is practiced will differ depending on the outcome you want from it, but an overarching definition of meditation is "a set of techniques that are intended to encourage a heightened state of awareness and focused attention" (Cherry, 2022). Meditation is also defined as being conscious-changing as you try to change your state of consciousness to improve your psychological well-being. Here are some of the most significant benefits you can get from meditation:

- **Mental health:** The mental health benefits of meditation have made it popular in Western society. Meditation is associated with increased focus, clarity, compassion, awareness, and calmness. Studies have also shown decreased symptoms of anxiety and depression, as high as a 46% reduction in depression and a 31% reduction in anxiety. People who meditate also can see an increase in mental resilience by 11% (Headspace, 2018).

- **Physical health:** Meditation is one of the best methods for coping with stress, and it allows us to learn how to calm the parasympathetic nervous system, which helps lower cortisol levels. A study of students meditating for ten days showed a 12% decrease in stress and an even bigger decrease in those who sustained meditation as a habit (Headspace, 2018). Meditation is also linked to reduced inflammation, decreasing your risk of heart disease, diabetes, cancer, and other diseases.
- **Gut health:** Meditation causes an increase in oxygen supply to our intestines which helps to improve digestion. The other mental and physical benefits that someone can get from meditating can also reduce other gastrointestinal symptoms, which are exacerbated by stress, not sleeping enough, or other health issues.

Meditation can get complicated for beginners, especially if you aren't using more advanced techniques. Here are some of the best meditation techniques for beginners:

- **Breathing meditation:** Use different breathing techniques to help calm the mind and reduce stress. The easiest breathing meditation for beginners is to sit down, close your eyes, breathe in through the nose, hold for a couple of seconds, and breathe out through the mouth. Repeat this for a few minutes.

- **Mantra meditation:** Combine breathing meditation with a mantra that you repeat as you breathe in or out.
- **Body scan meditation:** Keep your breathing calm, but also pay close attention to your bodily sensations.

If you are a beginner at meditation, here are some tips to try:

- **Set a schedule:** Meditate at the same time every day, whether this is before bed when you wake up, or any other time. Doing it consistently every day makes it easier to form a habit.
- **Get comfortable:** Being as comfortable as possible will make it much easier to fall into the right mindset for meditation.
- **Start slow:** You don't need to do a super long meditation session when you are first starting. Start slow and meditate only for a few minutes. As you grow more comfortable, meditate for longer.

- **Don't suppress your feelings; focus on them:** During meditation, your mind can wander, leading to you experiencing thoughts and feelings you find distressing or uncomfortable. It's important not to suppress these feelings; rather, allow yourself to acknowledge them and then let them go without judging yourself.

SLEEP

As we learned earlier in this book, sleep is essential to gut health. Let's recap its importance. When we sleep, our body goes through various cycles that allow for multiple processes to occur; some of these processes involve the production of microbiota, digestion of food, energy conservation, and many more. When we don't get enough sleep, the body can't go through these processes, leading to various health issues, including digestive issues. Sleep deprivation highly impacts our gut microbiota, causing imbalance, which can develop digestive diseases. Here are some sleep hacks for achieving sound sleep:

- **Stick to a sleep schedule:** You need seven to nine hours each night. Treat your sleep as work or an appointment, and block out nine hours you will dedicate to sleeping. Don't let anything interrupt this time. Make sure this schedule is the same every day.

- **Create a restful environment:** Your bedroom needs to be a place that promotes relaxation. Your bedroom should not make you feel stressed and should ease you into sleep. Keep the room cooler at night, disconnect from screens, keep the room dark, and block out noise.

- **Watch what you are eating and drinking before bed:** Alcohol and caffeine are the biggest enemies to sleep. Eating too close to bed can make it harder to fall asleep or stay asleep.

- **Manage your stress:** Resolve stress or any worries you have before bed. When stressed, you can start to ruminate while trying to sleep, making it much harder to fall asleep.

- **Limit your naps:** Naps during the day can make it harder to fall asleep at night. If you are going to take a nap, make sure it is not longer than 30 minutes, and earlier in the day rather than later.

- **Exercise regularly:** Physical activity helps to promote sleep through the release of hormones that energizes you throughout the day. However, don't exercise close to the bed, or it will keep you up.

The way that you wake up in the morning can have a significant impact on your day. If your wake-up patterns are jarring and sporadic, it can make it harder to create a routine, but it can also affect your mood and gut health, especially if your wake-up times differ significantly. Here are some tips to make waking up easier:

- **Wake up at a consistent time:** Waking up at the same time every day can significantly help with setting a sleep schedule as you will start to become tired at the same time every day. As you wake up consistently, your brain and body will begin to work like clockwork, and you will notice that you naturally start waking up at the same time, even without an alarm.
- **Meditate:** Meditating in the morning is a great way to cultivate success for the day, making it easier to cope with stress and pressure during the day and making it easier to fall asleep at night. Meditation is also a great way to allow yourself to wake up slowly instead of immediately hopping into the day.
- **Let the light in** Exposure to bright light during the day is great for your circadian rhythms, which will help you to fall asleep and wake up at the right times. Allowing for light in the

morning will also make it much easier to wake up.

TACKLING STRESS LEVELS

Stress is the silent killer, and it not only affects your gut health, but it will cause adverse reactions throughout all forms of health. People who are stressed are more likely to experience IBD, IBS, peptic ulcer disease, gastroesophageal reflux, and any form of gastrointestinal issues. Think of a time when you were stressed; you might have experienced heartburn, stomach pain, cramping, or other forms of gastrointestinal distress.

Stress can also impact other areas of health, including mental, emotional, and other physical health issues other than the gut, which can impact your gut health even more. You need to learn to tackle your stress levels, and luckily there are so many ways to do this. Here are some activities to try to reduce stress levels:

- **Breathing techniques:** It's incredible what just breathing can do to reduce your stress levels. Some breathing techniques to try include:
- **Deep breathing:** Stress often makes us take short quick breaths, which makes it harder to focus and increases feelings of anxiety. To practice deep breathing, you will lay on your

back and take deep breaths in and out, paying attention to how your stomach rises and falls with each breath.

- **Breath focus:** For this method, you are going to think of a word or phrase that calms you. After you have chosen one, close your eyes and breath deeply. Imagine your stress leaving as you breathe out and as you breathe in, think about the word or phrase that calms you. Do this for 10 minutes.

- **Progressive muscle relaxation:** Stress is associated with muscle tension, and relaxing these muscles can significantly reduce stress. To practice this, you will tighten a group of muscles as you breathe in and loosen them as you breathe out. Start from your toes and work your way up to your head.

- **Listen to music:** Listening to your favorite music can be a great way to get you out of your head and improve your mood.

- **Find the sun/practice "grounding":** Ground yourself by finding items that are a certain color, counting backward, or identifying your senses.

- **Hand or foot massage:** Both can help with tension caused by stress.

- **Get some alone time:** Sometimes having many people around can be overwhelming and adds to the stress. Getting some alone time is a great way to clear your mind.
- **Get organized:** Stress is often exacerbated by disorganization. Organizing your workspace is a great way to reduce stress.
- **Other activities:** Walking, yoga, stretching, working out, closing your eyes, and using a stress ball are all great outlets for stress.

Meditation, sleeping, and learning to cope with stress are essential habits for improving your gut health. It's important to remember that not every habit will work for you, but make sure to give everything a good try before disregarding it. We've reached the end of our journey, and you have learned all about the gut and the secret tips for improving your gut health. Before you start making healthy changes to your diet and lifestyle, let's recap what we have learned.

CONCLUSION

Gut health issues are some of the most common health issues that can be experienced, with women experiencing them much more often than men. Your gut is vital to all areas of your life, as it makes up 80% of your immune system and has a deep connection with the brain. This means that all areas of your health are intertwined. Making healthy changes in all areas of your life will benefit your gut health, and making changes to your gut health will positively impact your overall health.

Remember that to make your gut microbiota happy, you need to feed it the right things. But, your diet isn't the only change you need to make. Healthy habits such as meditating, exercising regularly, and getting enough sleep can improve your gut and overall health.

You've unlocked the door to a healthier gut, and regaining your health is now within your reach. Now it's time for you to take steps to make the changes you need to have a healthier life. You might experience setbacks in your life, but that does not mean you have failed and that you can't make these changes. Get back up and keep trying.

Please leave a review telling others how this book has helped you.

REFERENCES

Almekinder, E. (2019, April 25). *6 ways to improve gut health.* Blue Zones. https://www.bluezones.com/2019/04/6-ways-to-improve-gut-health/

American College of Gastroenterology. (n.d.). *Common GI problems in women.* American College of Gastroenterology. https://gi.org/topics/common-gi-problems-in-women/

Andrews, R. (2010, May 3). *All about probiotics: How to get them from both food and supplements.* Precision Nutrition. https://www.precisionnutrition.com/all-about-probiotics

Aubrey, A., & Godoy, M. (2016, August 3). 75 percent of Americans say they eat healthy, despite evidence to the contrary. *NPR.* https://www.npr.org/sections/thesalt/2016/08/03/487640479/75-percent-of-americans-say-they-eat-healthy-despite-evidence-to-the-contrary?t=1648463114925

Aubrey-Jones, D. (2020). *The cecum.* Teach Me Anatomy. https://teachmeanatomy.info/abdomen/gi-tract/cecum/

Aubrey-Jones, D. (2022, April 10). *The colon.* Teach Me Anatomy. https://teachmeanatomy.info/abdomen/gi-tract/colon/

Aziz-Scott, G. (2020, June 29). *Hormones & gut health: The estrobolome & hormone balance.* Marion Gluck. https://www.mariongluckclinic.com/blog/hormones-and-gut-health-the-estrobolome-and-hormone-balance.html

Batson, J. (2011). *What is stress?* The American Institute of Stress. https://www.stress.org/daily-life

Benefiber. (n.d.). *Why high fiber guts are good for gut health.* Benefiber. https://www.benefiber.com/amp/how-fiber-improves-gut-health.html

Benna, S. (2015). *The 6 everyday activities that are stressing you out.* Business Insider. https://www.businessinsider.com/everyday-activities-that-are-stressing-you-out-2015-8#2-relationships-2

Bolen, B. (2022). *How functional gastrointestinal disorders are diagnosed.* Verywell Health. https://www.verywellhealth.com/functional-gastrointestinal-disorders-1944874

Brazier, Y. (2017, December 15). *Celiac disease: Symptoms, diagnosis, diet, and treatment.* Medical News Today. https://www.medicalnewsto day.com/articles/38085

Brazier, Y. (2019, February 12). *Bacteria: Types, characteristics, where they live, hazards, and more.* Medical News Today. https://www.medical newstoday.com/articles/157973

Brighten The Brain. (2020). *What is digestion and how does the body rid itself of toxins?* Brighten the Brain. http://www.brightenthebrain. com/nutrition-and-detoxing-the-body/what-is-digestion-and-how-does-the-body-rid-itself-of-toxins

Carrie. (2019, December 27). *Grilled chicken thighs with pineapple-mint salsa.* 20 Dishes. https://www.20dishes.com/grilled-chicken-thighs-with-pineapple-mint-salsa/

Castaneda, R. (2022). *6 worst foods for gut health.* U.S. News Health. https://health.usnews.com/wellness/food/slideshows/worst-food-for-gut-health

Celiac Disease Foundation. (2017, December 31). *What is celiac disease?* Celiac Disease Foundation. https://celiac.org/about-celiac-disease/what-is-celiac-disease/

Chai, C. (2022). *Can a healthier gut microbiome boost mood?* Everyday Health. https://www.everydayhealth.com/emotional-health/can-a-healthier-gut-boost-your-mood/

Chatellier, C. (2021). *5 exercises that aid in optimal digestive health.* Gastroenterology HealthCare Associates. https://www.giwebmd. com/blog/2021/5/25/5-exercises-that-aid-in-optimal-digestive-health

Cherry, K. (2022). *How meditation impacts your mind and body.* Verywell Mind. https://www.verywellmind.com/what-is-meditation-2795927#toc-tips-for-meditating

Cleveland Clinic. (2015, December 31). *How gut bacteria may help curb your heart disease.* Cleveland Clinic. https://health.clevelandclinic. org/how-gut-bacteria-may-help-curb-heart-disease/#:~:

Cleveland Clinic. (2016). *Crohn's disease.* Cleveland Clinic. https://my. clevelandclinic.org/health/diseases/9357-crohns-disease

Cleveland Clinic. (2019). *Constipation.* Cleveland Clinic. https://my. clevelandclinic.org/health/diseases/4059-constipation

Cleveland Clinic. (2020a, February 5). *5 reasons you should add more fermented foods to your diet.* Cleveland Clinic. https://health.cleve landclinic.org/5-reasons-you-should-add-more-fermented-foods-to-your-diet-infographic/

Cleveland Clinic. (2020b, April 23). *Ulcerative colitis.* Cleveland Clinic. https://my.clevelandclinic.org/health/diseases/10351-ulcerative-colitis

Cleveland Clinic. (2020c, September 24). *Irritable bowel syndrome: IBS, symptoms, causes, treatment.* Cleveland Clinic. https://my.cleveland clinic.org/health/diseases/4342-irritable-bowel-syndrome-ibs

Cleveland Clinic. (2020d, December 10). *How to improve your digestive track naturally.* Cleveland Clinic. https://health.clevelandclinic.org/ how-to-improve-your-digestive-track-naturally/

Cleveland Clinic. (2021a). *Gastrointestinal diseases: Symptoms, treatment & causes.* Cleveland Clinic. https://my.clevelandclinic.org/health/ articles/7040-gastrointestinal-diseases

Cleveland Clinic. (2021b, August 9). *Digestive system: Function, organs and anatomy.* Cleveland Clinic. https://my.clevelandclinic.org/ health/body/7041-digestive-system

Coyle, D. (2017). *8 surprising things that harm your gut bacteria.* Health-line. https://www.healthline.com/nutrition/8-things-that-harm-gut-bacteria

Crawford, N. (2011, May 7). *How unhealthy foods affect the body.* Live-strong. https://www.livestrong.com/article/436610-how-unhealthy-foods-affect-the-body/

Crohn's and Colitis Foundation. (2019). *Causes of Crohn's disease.* Crohn's & Colitis Foundation. https://www.crohnscolitisfounda tion.org/what-is-crohns-disease/causes

Crosta, P. (2017, May 30). *Viruses: What are they and what do they do?* Medical News Today. https://www.medicalnewstoday.com/arti cles/158179

Danone Nutricia Research. (n.d.). *The central role of the gut.* Danone Nutricia Research. https://www.nutriciaresearch.com/gut-and-microbiology/the-central-role-of-the-gut/

Dix, M., & Klein, E. (2018). *7 signs of an unhealthy gut and 7 ways to improve gut health.* Healthline. https://www.healthline.com/health/gut-health#signs-and-symptoms

Drug.com. (n.d.). *Celiac disease (non-tropical sprue) Guide: Causes, symptoms and treatment options.* Drugs.com. https://www.drugs.com/health-guide/celiac-disease-non-tropical-sprue.html

Drugs.com. (n.d.). *Ulcerative colitis guide: Causes, symptoms and treatment options.* Drugs.com. https://www.drugs.com/health-guide/ulcerative-colitis.html

Drugs.com. (2019). *Constipation and impaction.* Drugs.com. https://www.drugs.com/health-guide/constipation-and-impaction.html

Dyckman, R. (2022). *5 surprising symptoms of an unhealthy gut.* Everyday Health. https://www.everydayhealth.com/digestive-health/surprising-symptoms-of-an-unhealthy-gut/

Eske, J. (2019, August 21). *Leaky gut syndrome: What it is, symptoms, and treatments.* Medical News Today. https://www.medicalnewstoday.com/articles/326117

Family Doctor Editorial Staff. (n.d.). *Constipation.* Family Doctor. https://familydoctor.org/condition/constipation/

Fields, H. (2014). *The gut: Where bacteria and immune system meet.* John Hopkins Medicine. https://www.hopkinsmedicine.org/research/advancements-in-research/fundamentals/in-depth/the-gut-where-bacteria-and-immune-system-meet

Fontenot, B. (2011, November 26). *Easy ways to incorporate more phytochemicals into your diet.* The Atlantic. https://www.theatlantic.com/health/archive/2011/11/easy-ways-to-incorporate-more-phytochemicals-into-your-diet/249012/

Foster, K. (2020). *Memorize this simple ratio for the best overnight oats.* Kitchen. https://www.thekitchn.com/overnight-oats-268370#post-recipe-13945

Fowler, P. (2018, January 11). *Breathing techniques for stress relief.* WebMD. https://www.webmd.com/balance/stress-management/stress-relief-breathing-techniques

Frederick Health. (2021). *10 signs of an unhealthy gut.* Frederick Health. https://www.frederickhealth.org/news/2021/july/10-signs-of-an-unhealthy-gut/

Gilbert Lab. (2020). *How your gut affects your immune system: A symbiotic relationship.* Gilbert Lab. https://gilbertlab.com/immune-system/gut-microbiome-symbiosis/

Gunnars, K. (2018, May 23). *Why is fiber good for you? The crunchy truth.* Healthline. https://www.healthline.com/nutrition/why-is-fiber-good-for-you

Harvard Health. (2018, July). *Fermented foods can add depth to your diet.* Harvard Health. https://www.health.harvard.edu/staying-healthy/fermented-foods-can-add-depth-to-your-diet

Harvard Health. (2019). *The gut-brain connection.* Harvard Health. https://www.health.harvard.edu/diseases-and-conditions/the-gut-brain-connection

Harvard T.H. Chan. (2019, September 4). *The microbiome.* The Nutrition Source. https://www.hsph.harvard.edu/nutritionsource/microbiome/

Headspace. (2018). *The many benefits of meditation.* Headspace. https://www.headspace.com/meditation/benefits

Headspace. (2020). *Wake up: How to wake up for non-morning people.* Headspace. https://www.headspace.com/sleep/how-to-wake-up-for-non-morning-people

Henry Ford Health Staff. (2021). *How lack of sleep can affect gut health.* Henry Ford Health. https://www.henryford.com/blog/2021/02/sleep-affects-gut-health

Hickman, K. (2021, September 14). *Ugly side effects of the american diet, say dietitians.* Eat This Not That. https://www.eatthis.com/ugly-side-effects-american-diet/

Hill, C., Guarner, F., Reid, G., Gibson, G. R., Merenstein, D. J., Pot, B., Morelli, L., Canani, R. B., Flint, H. J., Salminen, S., Calder, P. C., & Sanders, M. E. (2014). The international scientific association for probiotics and prebiotics consensus statement on the scope and appropriate use of the term probiotic. *Nature Reviews. Gastroenterology & Hepatology, 11*(8), 506–514. https://doi.org/10.1038/nrgastro.2014.66

Huizen, J. (2020, December 24). *How gut microbes contribute to good sleep.* Medical News Today. https://www.medicalnewstoday.com/articles/how-gut-microbes-contribute-to-good-sleep#Conducting-the-study

Johns Hopkins Medicine. (n.d.-a). *5 foods to avoid if you have IBS.* Johns Hopkins Medicine. https://www.hopkinsmedicine.org/health/conditions-and-diseases/irritable-bowel-syndrome-ibs/5-foods-to-avoid-if-you-have-ibs

Johns Hopkins Medicine. (n.d.-b). *Constipation.* Johns Hopkins Medicine. https://www.hopkinsmedicine.org/health/conditions-and-diseases/constipation

Jones, O. (2012). *The small intestine.* Teach Me Anatomy. https://teachmeanatomy.info/abdomen/gi-tract/small-intestine/

Jones, O. (2018, December 10). *The appendix.* Teach Me Anatomy. https://teachmeanatomy.info/abdomen/gi-tract/appendix/

Kingsland, J. (2022, February 1). *Long COVID: Gut bacteria may be key.* Www.medicalnewstoday.com. https://www.medicalnewstoday.com/articles/gut-bacteria-may-play-a-role-in-the-development-of-long-covid#Potential-treatments

Klein, S. L., & Flanagan, K. L. (2016). Sex differences in immune responses. *Nature Reviews Immunology, 16*(10), 626–638. https://doi.org/10.1038/nri.2016.90

Koziol, M. (2015, April 9). *The 10 everyday things we stress over.* The Sydney Morning Herald. https://www.smh.com.au/lifestyle/the-10-everyday-things-we-stress-over-20150408-1mgknb.html

Lankeneu Medical Centre. (2017, May 3). *Medications that can impact your gut health.* Main Line Health. https://www.mainlinehealth.org/blog/medications-and-gut-health

Laurence, E. (2017, January 30). *Why women have more digestive problems than men.* Well+Good. https://www.wellandgood.com/why-women-have-more-gut-problems/

Laurence, E. (2021, January 21). *4 ways gut health affects sleep.* Well+Good. https://www.wellandgood.com/gut-health-affects-sleep/

Lee, L. (2019). *5 foods to improve your digestion.* Johns Hopkins Medicine. https://www.hopkinsmedicine.org/health/wellness-and-preven tion/5-foods-to-improve-your-digestion

Lewis, S. (2020, September 9). *Probiotics and prebiotics: What's the differ-ence?* Healthline. https://www.healthline.com/nutrition/probiotics-and-prebiotics#whats-the-difference

MacGill, M. (2018, June 26). *Gut microbiota: Definition, importance, and medical uses.* Medical News Today. https://www.medicalnewstoday. com/articles/307998

Maimonides. (n.d.). *Maimonides quotes.* Brainy Quote. https://www. brainyquote.com/quotes/maimonides_326756

Mahmood, H. (2016). *The anal canal.* Teach Me Anatomy. https://teach meanatomy.info/abdomen/gi-tract/anal-canal/

Makowska, K., & Gonkowski, S. (2019). Age and Sex-Dependent Differences in the Neurochemical Characterization of Calcitonin Gene-Related Peptide-Like Immunoreactive (CGRP-LI) Nervous Structures in the Porcine Descending Colon. *International Journal of Molecular Sciences, 20*(5), 1024. https://doi.org/10.3390/ ijms20051024

Manaker, L. (2021). *How does deep breathing improve your digestion?* Very-well Health. https://www.verywellhealth.com/diaphragmatic-breathing-stress-digestion-5209648

Mathews, N. (2014). *The esophagus.* Teach Me Anatomy. https://teach meanatomy.info/abdomen/gi-tract/oesophagus/

Mayfair Diagnostics. (2019). *How does the gastrointestinal system change with age?* Radiology. https://www.radiology.ca/article/how-does-gastrointestinal-system-change-age

Mayo Clinic. (2020, October 13). *Crohn's disease: Symptoms and causes.* Mayo Clinic. https://www.mayoclinic.org/diseases-conditions/crohns-disease/symptoms-causes/syc-20353304

Mayo Clinic Staff. (2018). *Irritable bowel syndrome: Symptoms and causes.* Mayo Clinic. https://www.mayoclinic.org/diseases-conditions/irritable-bowel-syndrome/symptoms-causes/syc-20360016

Mayo Clinic Staff. (2020, April 17). *6 steps to better sleep.* Mayo Clinic. https://www.mayoclinic.org/healthy-lifestyle/adult-health/in-depth/sleep/art-20048379

McCoy, K. (2017, August 24). *10 tips for better digestive health.* Everyday Health. https://www.everydayhealth.com/digestive-health/tips-for-better-digestive-health/

McMillen, M. (2011, July 12). *Leaky gut syndrome: What is it?* WebMD. https://www.webmd.com/digestive-disorders/features/leaky-gut-syndrome

Meridian Chiropractic Health Center. (2018, March 3). *What are postbiotics? 5 health benefits.* Meridian Chiropractic Health Center. https://www.chiropractor-schaumburg.com/what-are-postbiotics-5-health-benefits/

Microbiology Society. (2021). *Bacteria.* Microbiology Society. https://microbiologysociety.org/why-microbiology-matters/what-is-microbiology/bacteria.html

Migala, J. (2021). *Low-FODMAP diet guide: Complete scientific guide.* Everyday Health. https://www.everydayhealth.com/diet-nutrition/low-fodmap-diet/

Mind. (2017, November). *Causes of stress.* Www.mind.org.uk. https://www.mind.org.uk/information-support/types-of-mental-health-problems/stress/causes-of-stress/

Mindful. (2019, April 13). *How to meditate.* Mindful. https://www.mindful.org/how-to-meditate/

Minimalist Baker. (2014, April 8). *Vegan garlic pasta.* Minimalist Baker. https://minimalistbaker.com/creamy-vegan-garlic-pasta-with-roasted-tomatoes/

Naidoo, U. (2019, March 27). *Gut feelings: How food affects your mood.* Harvard Health. https://www.health.harvard.edu/blog/gut-feelings-how-food-affects-your-mood-2018120715548

NHS. (2019, January 23). *Overview: Ulcerative colitis.* NHS. https://www.nhs.uk/conditions/ulcerative-colitis/

Nourished by Nutrition. (2019, March 28). *7 unexpected things messing with your gut bacteria.* Nourished by Nutrition. https://nourishedbynutrition.com/7-unexpected-things-messing-with-your-gut-bacteria/

Patino, E. (2020). *Signs of an unhealthy gut and what you can do about it.* Everyday Health. https://www.everydayhealth.com/digestive-health/signs-of-unhealthy-gut-and-how-to-fix-it/

Pedre, V. (2018, June 29). *Poor gut health will mess with this hormone.* MBGHealth. https://www.mindbodygreen.com/articles/poor-gut-health-will-mess-with-this-hormone

Pesheva, E. (2021). *Diet, gut microbes, and immunity.* Harvard Medical School. https://hms.harvard.edu/news/diet-gut-microbes-immunity

Pratt, E. (2018, January 12). *Exercise and gut bacteria.* Healthline. https://www.healthline.com/health-news/exercise-improves-your-gut-bacteria

Pritikin. (n.d.). *The typical American diet is our biggest enemy.* Pritikin. https://www.pritikin.com/your-health/healthy-living/eating-right/1789-american-diet-our-biggest-risk-factor-for-disease-disability-and-death.html

Psychologies. (2022, April 19). *Gut health diet: Your 4-week meal plan.* Psychologies. https://www.psychologies.co.uk/gut-health-diet/

Raman, R. (2017, July 2). *How to do an elimination diet and why.* Healthline. https://www.healthline.com/nutrition/elimination-diet

Raman, R. (2021, May 19). *What are postbiotics? Types, benefits, and downsides.* Healthline. https://www.healthline.com/nutrition/postbiotics

Renew Life Probiotics. (2016). *New study reveals women may suffer from digestive health issues in silence.* Cision PR Newswire. https://www.prnewswire.com/news-releases/new-study-reveals-women-may-suffer-from-digestive-health-issues-in-silence-300373970.html

Robertson, R. (2017, June 27). *Why the gut microbiome is crucial for your health.* Healthline. https://www.healthline.com/nutrition/gut-microbiome-and-health#TOC_TITLE_HDR_2

Roswell Park Comprehensive Cancer Center. (2019). *For the health benefits of phytochemicals, "eat a rainbow."* Roswell Park Comprehensive Cancer Center. https://www.roswellpark.org/cancertalk/201912/health-benefits-phytochemicals-eat-rainbow

Scott, L. A. (n.d.). *Gut health and hormones.* Achieve Optimal Wellness. https://www.leighannscottmd.com/additional-testing/gut-health-and-hormones/

Shiraz, Z. (2021, November 28). *Yoga for gut health: 5 exercises to aid in digestion, reset your system.* Hindustan Times. https://www.hindustantimes.com/lifestyle/health/yoga-for-gut-health-5-exercises-to-aid-in-digestion-reset-your-system-101638096143638.html

Sissons, C. (2019, July 23). *How to improve digestion: Tips and tricks.* Medical News Today. https://www.medicalnewstoday.com/articles/325822

Smith, J. (2021). *Celiac disease: Symptoms, diagnosis, diet, and treatment.* Medical News Today. https://www.medicalnewstoday.com/articles/38085#causes

Spritzler, F. (2016). *21 reasons to eat real food.* Healthline. https://www.healthline.com/nutrition/21-reasons-to-eat-real-food

Stephens, H. (n.d.). *The effects of an American diet on health.* UAB. https://www.uab.edu/inquiro/issues/past-issues/volume-9/the-effects-of-an-american-diet-on-health

Thaichon, P., & Quach, S. (2015). *How marketers condition us to buy more junk food.* The Conversation. https://theconversation.com/how-marketers-condition-us-to-buy-more-junk-food-43466

The Gut Choice. (2021, February 13). *7 at-home workouts to boost your gut health.* The Gut Choice. https://thegutchoice.com/2021/02/13/7-at-home-workouts-to-boost-your-gut-health-tried-tested/

Theakston, V. (2018). *The rectum.* Teach Me Anatomy. https://teachmeanatomy.info/abdomen/gi-tract/rectum/

TNN. (2015). *Here's how to make your kitchen diet-friendly.* The Times of India. https://timesofindia.indiatimes.com/life-style/health-fitness/weight-loss/heres-how-to-make-your-kitchen-diet-friendly/articleshow/31675086.cms

Unicef. (2021). *Marketing of unhealthy foods and non-alcoholic beverages to children* (pp. 1–19). https://www.unicef.org/media/116691/file/Marketing%20restrictions.pdf

Valdes, A. M., Walter, J., Segal, E., & Spector, T. D. (2018). Role of the gut microbiota in nutrition and health. *BMJ, 361*(361), k2179. https://doi.org/10.1136/bmj.k2179

Veloso, H. (n.d.). *FODMAP diet: What you need to know.* Johns Hopkins Medicine. https://www.hopkinsmedicine.org/health/wellness-and-prevention/fodmap-diet-what-you-need-to-know

Vizthum, D. (2019). *5 spices with healthy benefits.* Johns Hopkins Medicine. https://www.hopkinsmedicine.org/health/wellness-and-prevention/5-spices-with-healthy-benefits

Voigt, R. M., Forsyth, C. B., Green, S. J., Mutlu, E., Engen, P., Vitaterna, M. H., Turek, F. W., & Keshavarzian, A. (2014). Circadian disorganization alters intestinal microbiota. *PLoS ONE, 9*(5), e97500. https://doi.org/10.1371/journal.pone.0097500

Walker, D. (2013). *The stomach.* Teach Me Anatomy. https://teachmeanatomy.info/abdomen/gi-tract/stomach/

Watson, S., & Cherney, K. (2020, May 15). *11 effects of sleep deprivation on your body.* Healthline. https://www.healthline.com/health/sleep-deprivation/effects-on-body#Causes-of-sleep-deprivation

WebMD. (n.d.). *Super steps to boost digestive health.* WebMD. https://www.webmd.com/digestive-disorders/ss/slideshow-digestion-tips

WebMD. (2019). *Types of yeast: Powerful little fungus.* WebMD. https://www.webmd.com/diet/ss/slideshow-yeast-and-your-body

Well+Good Editors. (2019, April 5). *This is what a week of workouts should look like if you want to optimize your gut health.* Well+Good. https://www.wellandgood.com/digestive-health-exercise-renew-life/

Zorfass, N. (2021, January 21). *Four exercises to support your gut microbiome*. Institute for Integrative Nutrition. https://www.integra tivenutrition.com/blog/four-exercises-to-support-your-gut-microbiome

Made in the USA
Las Vegas, NV
11 November 2023

80615526R00118